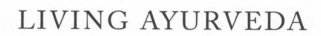

LIVING AYURVEDA

This book is dedicated
to the curious explorer within us all,
may we know our true nature . . .

LIVING AYURVEDA

Nourishing body and mind through
seasonal recipes, rituals, and yoga

Claire Ragozzino

ROOST BOOKS

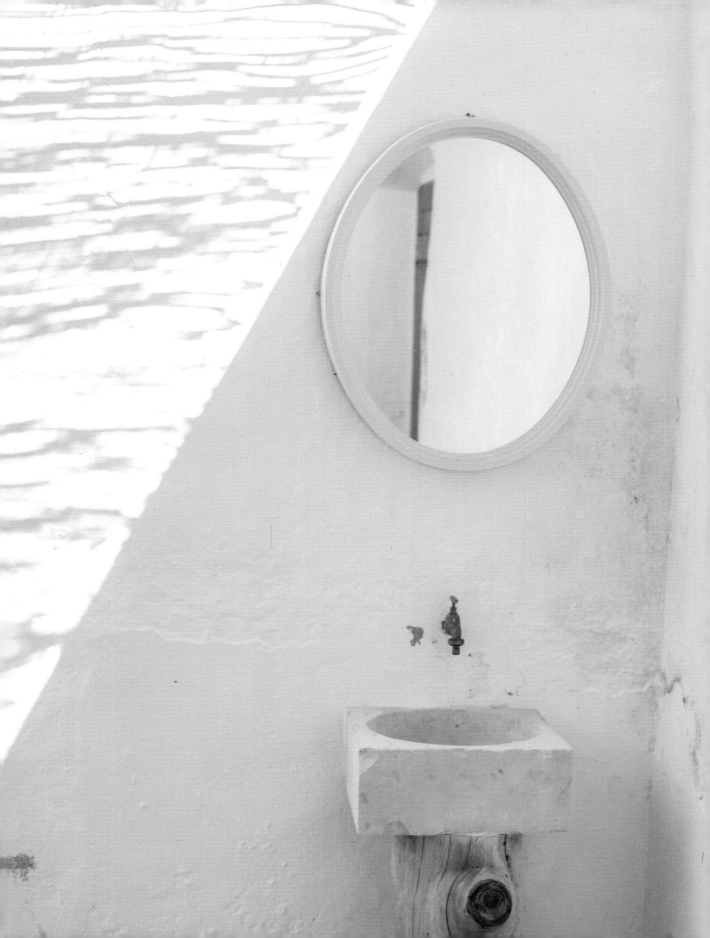

CONTENTS

INTRODUCTION

I first discovered Ayurveda during my own healing crisis. I was struggling with a chronic digestive disorder that doctors couldn't figure out. Searching for answers, I tried every diet, cleanse, supplement, and superfood under the sun. I saw all kinds of specialists and healers. I read and researched everything I could find, spending my days absorbed in the pages of every holistic health book I could get my hands on. Each nugget of knowledge felt like a bread crumb trail leading more closer to what I was seeking. Then, I came across Dr. Vasant Lad's primer, *Ayurveda: The Science of Self-Healing*, and a spark ignited within me. The concept of viewing the body-mind-soul as an intelligent whole couldn't have felt more right. And in a sea of information on trendy diets and health hacks, this wisdom felt timeless and true for me in a way nothing else had before.

I'll admit, at first I found the Sanskrit words and the concepts foreign. The more I studied, the more complicated it all felt. As I approached learning Ayurveda from my head, the lists of what I should and shouldn't eat for my body type grew even more confusing. I turned to an Ayurvedic practitioner for guidance, and the best advice I received was to stop studying and take a year to discover this wisdom for myself, at my own pace. So that's just what I did, and it changed my life.

I took the year to first explore food and create more mindfulness around *how* I was eating, not just *what* I was eating. This simple shift alone had a huge impact on my digestion. Then I turned to yoga, looking to experience why different sequences were more supportive for me at different times of the year and cycles in my life. I established a regular routine, something I hadn't previously had, and gave myself space to be a curious observer of how these shifts in my daily lifestyle impacted my body and influenced my mind. I discovered that nourishment comes in many forms—the food we eat, the company we keep, the way we move our bodies and breathe, and how we create space each day for greater presence in our lives. Real nourishment, real self-care, is about taking time to pause for rituals that honor the ebb and flow of life's cycles. By learning to live by these cycles and rhythms, a deeper wisdom blossomed within me and my struggles with eating fell away as this new way of living emerged.

At the heart of it, this wisdom taught me how to have a different, more meaningful, relationship to time. In this hyper-stimulated culture we live in, there's always a sense of urgency and a pervasive notion of busyness. We fill our time with long lists of tasks and work late into the night to get them done, only to get up the next morning and do it all again. This unsustainable pace of modern life can create further disconnection from ourselves and nature, and this is where disease emerges. When our attention is pushed and pulled in a thousand directions at any given moment, how can we expect to know ourselves or understand our role in the natural world?

I believe it's more important than ever that we use these tools of awareness to reconnect with what's real. Ayurveda is not a fad or a trend; it's a time-tested science that applies to all cultures, places, and stages of life. If we slow down enough and learn how to listen, the answers to vibrant health and more empowered living can be found all around us.

This is my hope for you: Give yourself space and time to explore and experience this wisdom for yourself. What do the elements look like in your body? How does cooking with presence and intention through the seasons shift your relationship to food? What does it feel like to live by the rhythms of nature guiding your life? There is no right or wrong here, simply a practice of self-observation without judgment.

This book—part cookbook, part lifestyle guide—is meant to be a home-practice manual for your daily self-exploration. It takes you through the arc of a year, exploring how to use food, breath, movement, meditation, and ritual to connect you to the seasons. In part one, you'll uncover the language of Ayurveda—from understanding the elements to looking at the daily and seasonal cycles of nature—and how it influences your life. In part two, you'll prepare for your year, stocking your pantry with staples and creating sacred space in your home. And in part three, you'll dive into the seasons to explore different recipes, rituals, and yoga practices that nurture, balance, and nourish your well-being through the year.

I hope that this book sparks your curiosity for a different way of living. Let the kitchen and your yoga mat become a laboratory for self-study. Get to know yourself intimately, be open to new discoveries, and see where this path takes you. . . .

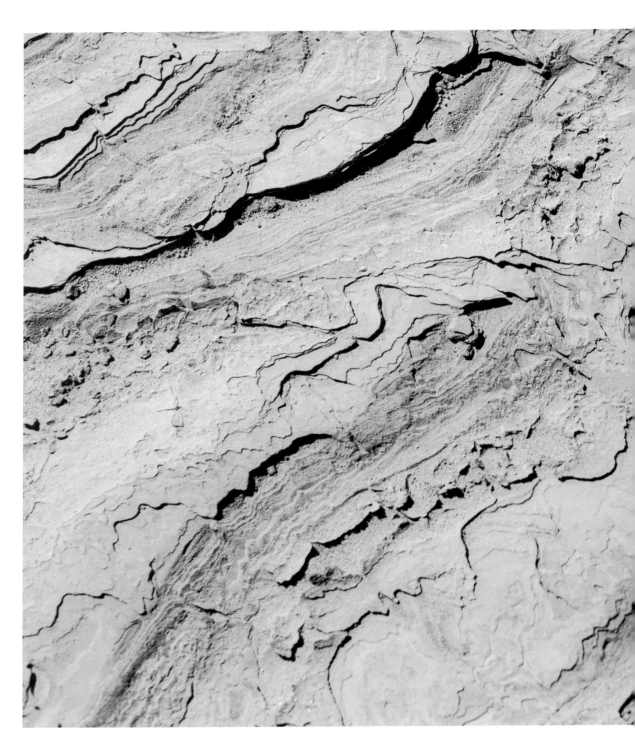

PART ONE

THE FOUNDATIONS OF

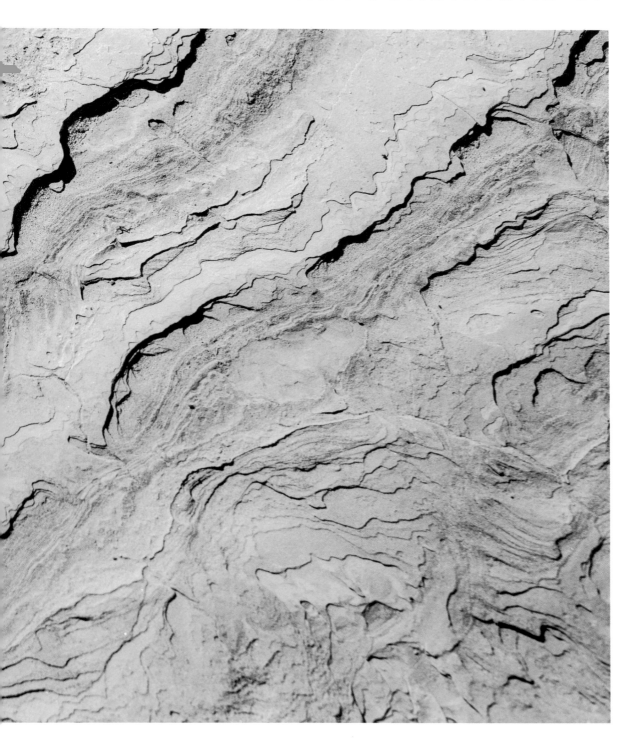

AYURVEDA

INTERPRETING THE LANGUAGE OF AYURVEDA

What is Ayurveda and how can you begin to make sense of this wisdom? I like to think of Ayurveda as a language that helps us describe the natural world and our relationship to it. I remember living in Paris and trying to learn French. At first, the language was difficult to grasp and translate. Then I started taking yoga classes at a nearby studio. I knew what the different parts of the body and breath were in the yoga sequences, so learning French became more intuitive when I applied it to my own physical experience. Over time, my comprehension expanded and soon I could speak more fluently. This is how I recommend approaching Ayurveda—taking the information slowly, not getting too heady with it or hung up on the Sanskrit words themselves, and instead looking at the ways you can identify the qualities of the elements and the doshas in your own body and mind. Over time, these concepts will become second nature—a cultivated intuition you'll learn to trust through your own direct experience.

Ayurveda is the indigenous medical system of India that views health through an all-encompassing lens, looking at the body-mind-spirit in relationship to nature. *Ayurveda* means "the knowledge of life and longevity," or another translation I enjoy, "the art of living." As poetic as this sounds, the roots of Ayurveda are deeply established in centuries of oral and written lineages of practiced medical science, with eight branches of specialties—general medicine; pediatrics; psychiatry; diseases of the head, neck, and face; surgery; toxicology; geriatrics/rejuvenation; and fertility/reproductive science. These eight limbs work together to support our health at different times of need, using both preventative and curative methods to nurture well-being through all stages of life. In India today, you'll find traditional Ayurvedic physicians (*vaidyas*) with community-based practices and Ayurvedic hospitals that work in tandem with Western medicine to provide holistic care. And around the world, Ayurvedic knowledge is growing widely as an empowering system for personal health and wellness through everyday self-care.

The word for "health" in Ayurveda is *svastha*. You know those people who radiate joy and literally glow? There's a juicy aliveness about them that is palpable and magnetic. This is svastha embodied—people who are confidently established in themselves. Our health isn't just the absence of disease; it's a dynamic state of harmony between our physical body, our mind, our senses, and our soul. Ayurveda teaches us how to care for these four aspects by paying close attention to the ways our surrounding environments affect our state of health, and how to use right thinking, diet, and lifestyle to maintain an inner equilibrium. This book seeks to empower you with knowledge and tools for becoming more firmly established in yourself, using food, breath, movement and meditation in harmony with nature's rhythms.

THE FIVE ELEMENTS

Ayurveda's core view is the connection between the macrocosm and the microcosm, from the universal to the individual, meaning what exists outside also exists within us. The five great elements (*pancha mahabhuta*) that compose the world around us also make up our inner world. These elements—space, air, fire, water, earth—form the building blocks of life and mirror the basic principles in physics of space, energy, transformation, liquid, and matter. Each element is connected to a subtle energy, a *tanmatra*, that is associated with our senses—sound, touch, vision, taste, and smell. Let's explore how the elements form our physical body.

Ether/Space (*Akasha*)

Ether or space, *akasha*, is the first and subtlest of all the elements. Ether is the space in which everything exists. It is universal, nonmoving, and formless. Its qualities are clear, light, subtle, soft, and immeasurable. This element is related to the actions of expansion and vibration. The tanmatra of space is sound (*shabda*), and the ear is the sensory organ that perceives sound.

Air (*Vayu*)

The air element, *vayu*, is the energy of movement. It initiates and directs motion. Its qualities are mobile, dry, light, cold, rough, and subtle. The tanmatra of air is touch (*sparsha*), and the sensory organ is skin, which helps detect movement. In the body, air expresses itself in the movement of the muscles, lungs, heart, and impulses of the nervous system. It's responsible for breathing, ingestion and elimination, and the flow of thought. *Prana* is the basic principle of the air element, the vital life force that is primarily taken in through breath and which life cannot exist without.

Fire (*Agni*)

The fire element, *agni*, is the energy of transformation. The qualities of fire are hot, sharp, light, dry, and subtle. The tanmatra of fire is vision (*rupa*), and the eyes are the sensory organ responsible for sight. The fire element governs all metabolic processes, aiding in the digestion of food, transformation of thoughts, and perception of light. *Tejas* is the subtle essence of fire, the burning flame of pure intelligence that processes all perception into knowledge.

Water (*Apas*)

From subtle to gross, the next element is water, called *apas*. Its main actions are cohesion and adhesion. Its qualities are cool, liquid, dull, soft, oily, and slimy. The tanmatra of water is taste (*rasa*). The tongue is the sensory organ that plays a large role in our experience of eating and our sense of satisfaction. Water lives in the body as plasma, saliva, mucous, cerebrospinal fluid, urine, and sweat. *Ojas* is the subtle essence of water, giving vitality and immunity to the bodily tissues.

Earth (*Prithvi*)

The earth element, *prithvi*, is the densest of all. It creates shape and structure. It is heavy, dull, dense, hard, and gross. The tanmatra of earth is smell (*gandha*), and the sensory organ is the nose. The earth element shapes all the body's solid structures and tissues, including the bones, cartilage, nails, teeth, hair, and skin.

THE TWENTY QUALITIES

The qualities that described each element, can also be used to describe everything in the manifest universe. These twenty qualities or ten pairs of opposites, known as the *gunas*, are particularly helpful in our personal practice because they provide a language that helps us identify our experience of the outside world and how it affects our inner world. These qualities can also be divided into two categories: those that are building (*brahmana*) and those that are lightening (*langhana*). Vata and pitta share the qualities of lightness, and kapha carries the opposing heaviness. This concept is much like the yin-yang principle in Chinese medicine.

Building		Lightening
Heavy	—	Light
Slow	—	Sharp
Cold	—	Hot
Oily	—	Dry
Smooth	—	Rough
Dense	—	Liquid
Soft	—	Hard
Stable	—	Mobile
Gross	—	Subtle
Cloudy	—	Clear

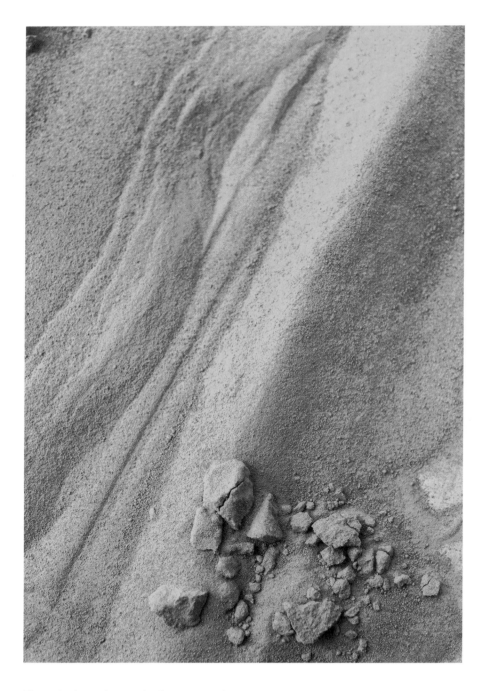

The whole universe is the expansion
of one's consciousness.

—*CARAKA SAMHITA*, SHARIRASTHANA 5,20

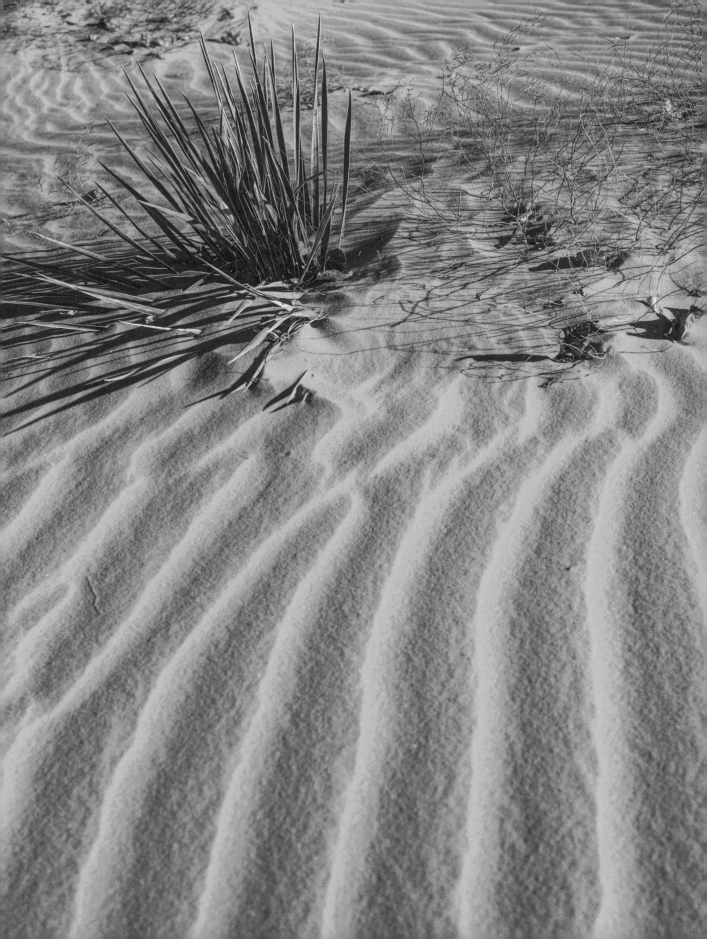

Knowing these qualities can help us identify how to bring balance into our lives. For example, if it's a hot summer and we regularly eat foods that are spicy and heating, we might experience more heat internally. Because like increases like, we can choose an activity or a diet that has the opposite quality to bring balance and support to our system.

THE DOSHAS

Ayurveda further groups these five elements into three energies or forces known as *doshas*—*vata*, *pitta*, *kapha*—which can be observed in everything from the seasons, to the time of day, to our own body type, and the functions within the body. Each dosha is a synergy of two elements. You can apply the twenty qualities to describe the doshas:

Vata = dry, light, cold, rough, subtle, mobile, clear

Pitta = oily, sharp, hot, light, mobile, liquid

Kapha = heavy, slow, cold, oily, liquid, smooth, dense, soft, stable, cloudy

Identifying the doshas and their qualities in your own body is the first step to understanding them and how they function.

Vata (Air + Space)

Vata is the energy of movement. Vata is the most mobile of the three doshas, and it initiates the movement of pitta and kapha, which are immobile. Thus it's the most unstable. When out of balance, vata can disturb the other doshas. Vata governs our nervous system, intellect, hearing, elimination, and all movement in our body's systems. It's located in the colon, pelvic cavity, lower back, thighs, bones, ears, skin, and nervous system.

Pitta (Fire + Water)

Pitta is the energy of transformation. The principle of fire governs metabolism and all the biochemical changes in our body, including digestion and temperature regulation. It helps us to digest everything we take in and make use of, from food to sensory input. It shapes our intelligence and discernment. Pitta is located in the small intestine, liver, spleen, gall bladder, blood, sweat, eyes, and endocrine glands.

Kapha (Water + Earth)

Kapha is the energy of stability, structure, and lubrication. Kapha governs the structural system and waterways of our body. It promotes anabolism, the process of building up the body and creating or repairing new cells. Kapha is located in the stomach, mucous membranes, plasma and lymph, cytoplasm in cells, white matter in brain, synovial fluid in joints, subcutaneous fat, mouth, nose, and all bodily secretions.

YOUR UNIQUE CONSTITUTION

While all three doshas—vata (V), pitta (P), kapha (K)—work to govern the different systems of our bodies, the proportion of each varies from person to person. Just as we have our own unique fingerprint, we each have our own unique constitutional makeup, known as *prakriti*. Prakriti is your birth constitution that shapes how you'll relate to your environment. A series of factors influence your birth constitution—from your parents' genetics and doshic imbalances at the time of conception to the type of diet your mother ate, what your birth experience was like, and your early childhood imprints. There are seven main combinations of constitutional types: V, P, K, VP, PK, VK, VPK. In some cases, though rare, all three doshas are equal in quality and quantity. Most of us will have one or two doshas present, with one dominant and the other secondary. Take a look at the primary types and how they manifest in the body and personality:

Vata Types

Vata types tend to have slender, narrow frames that are either very tall and lanky, or very short and petite. Their joints are prominent, their hair is darker, and their nails are dry or brittle. They have dark or pale complexions and their skin can be dry, rough, and cold. Their eyes are dark and sometimes small or sunken. Their hands and feet are often cold. Their appetite is often weak or variable, and their elimination can be scanty, irregular, and tending toward dryness or constipation. Keeping weight on is often a challenge. Vata types are quick learners and have great short-term memory but can have difficulty retaining information long-term. They are highly creative, visionary, and alert, but can tire easily or have trouble finishing a task before starting a new one. It can be difficult for vata types to stick to any kind of routine or daily ritual. Yet, they can benefit the most from having the stability of a regular routine.

Pitta Types

Pitta types have a medium and muscular build, they're not overly thin or overweight. They tend to run very warm and their skin is red or flushed. Their complexion is often coppery or yellow, fair, and freckled. Their eyes are green, gray, or coppery brown, and have a brightness or sharpness to them. Their hair can be fine, light brown, blonde, or red in color, and their nails are softer. Their appetite is insatiable, and their digestion is strong when protected. Their elimination is frequent and can be loose or liquid. They can gain or lose weight quickly. Pitta types are very intelligent, sharp thinkers and speakers, and quick learners. Their natural charisma, drive, and discipline makes them great leaders. But their excessive ambition can lead

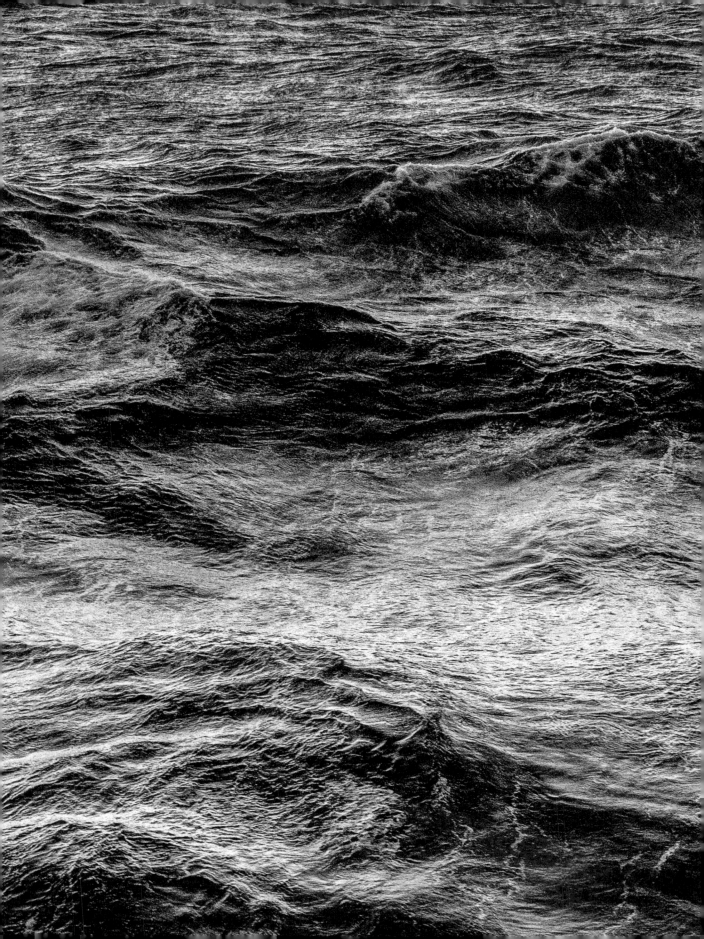

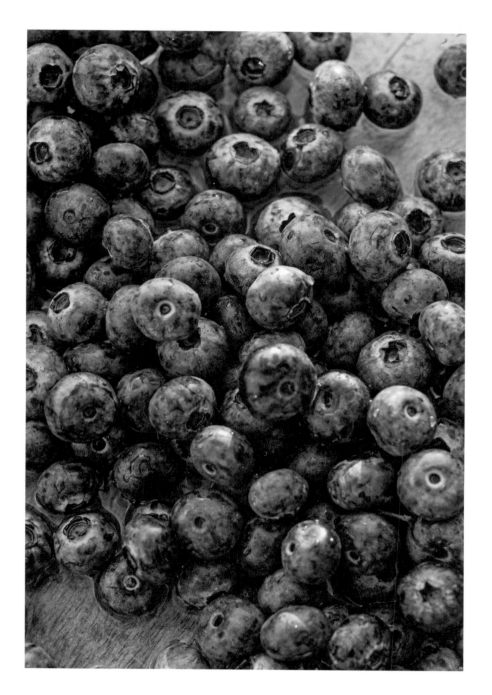

Vision is food for the eyes.
Sound is food for the ears.
Touch is food for the skin.
Taste is food for the tongue.

—DR. VASANT LAD

to habits of overworking and generally overdoing it to the point of burnout. A pitta type can thrive when they keep their intensity in check so as not to aggravate their already strong inner fire.

Kapha Types

Kapha types have a medium to broad frame with a larger bone structure and broad hips. Their bodies are well proportioned and sturdy, often with deep-set joints that are well-lubricated. Their skin and hair are thick, soft and oily, and their nails are strong. Their eyes are large and their lips very full. They have a regular appetite but tend toward slower digestion and elimination. It can be easy to gain weight and difficult to lose it. A kapha type has steady energy, good stamina, and a slow and calm disposition. It may take longer to learn new things and adapt to change, but when they do, their long-term memory is strong and their commitment unwavering. They are inherently loving, caring, generous, and kind. Habits and routines are easily formed and stuck to, but this can lead to rigidity and attachment if not careful.

YOUR PRESENT CONDITION

As you read through these main types, you might feel that you relate more to one over another. Or you may relate more to the physical characteristics of one and the mental characteristics of another. An online quiz can be a fun way to begin to explore the doshas, but the best way to determine your prakriti is to work with a trained practitioner who can identify this for you. I have listed several centers, schools, and online references in the resources section. Understanding your prakriti will better equip you with the right knowledge of your body-mind tendencies. For example, if you identified more with the vata qualities described above, you might be more easily influenced by a windy, cold day than someone with more pitta or kapha in their constitution. Prakriti is also the reason my friend and I can sit down at the dinner table to enjoy the same meal but have completely different experiences with how we digest the food and how the food impacts our inner world. Knowing our individual prakriti helps us understand our proclivities—why we favor certain foods and activities over others, and how nature's seasonal influences will uniquely affect our body and mind. It helps us know ourselves better and what actions we need to take to keep us in balance.

But before you get too caught up with identifying yourself ("I'm vata," "I'm pitta," "I'm kapha," etc.), take a step back and remember that you are composed of all the elements working in a harmonious, interdependent union within you. Prakriti is important, but it is not everything.

I remember reading dozens of Ayurvedic textbooks and feeling dizzy at first from all the information. Trying to make sense of it, I clung to all the charts for vata types. I tried to follow verbatim everything I should eat or do, and fervently avoid anything that was "bad" for me. This was helpful only for a short while, until the season shifted and so did my needs. By summer I was burning up and feeling bogged down by all the heavy, oily cooked foods that had fit so well in fall and winter. When we attach ourselves to one static idea of who we think we are or what diet we need, we miss out on the beauty behind Ayurveda's wisdom—the wisdom of awareness. Learning how our body types are affected by the seasons, the times of day, and the different cycles of life is key to maintaining that inner balance that shapes our health. This is where *vikriti* comes into play.

Our vikriti is our current state or present condition, the elemental makeup of our body's relationship to our current environment. Vikriti requires us to pay attention and stay present. When we notice in the peak of summer that we're feeling hot, agitated, and sharp, we can observe that pitta is high. Or if we are cold, our skin is dry, and our joints are popping, vata is high. If we feel sluggish, lethargic, or have a runny nose, kapha is high. These simple observations of how we feel in the moment help us identify imbalances and inform what action we should take to bring us back into balance. You don't need a dosha quiz to tell you if you're feeling hot or cold, heavy, or light. This is perhaps the most important tool in your home practice, and why I've based the whole structure of this book around creating a present-moment relationship with yourself and staying connected to the seasons and cycles of life.

Self-Inquiry

Determining what you need each day can be as simple as tuning in and observing what is present in your bodies and minds. Self-inquiry is a powerful tool to get to know yourself on physical, mental, and spiritual level. When you wake up in the morning, try asking yourself these two simple questions:

> *1. What is present today?* Observe how you're feeling in your body. Observe the quality of your thoughts and emotions.
>
> *2. What is needed?* What can you do to nourish you and bring you into balance today?

The Power of the Mind: The Maha Gunas

Remember, our health includes more than just tending to the physical body, it also requires us to understand our mind. Where the twenty qualities (*gunas*) are used primarily to describe the characteristics of the physical body and the material world around us, the *maha gunas* can describe the different expressions of our mind. The three maha gunas—*sattva*, *rajas*, and *tamas*—help us identify when we're in a state of clear and balanced thinking, when we're overactive or agitated, or when we're underactive or withdrawn.

Sattva means "light"; it's that state of clarity, illumination, harmony, and contentment. It's the feeling when all is right in the world and there's a sense of deep ease within. It's that calm, clear feeling we experience after a beautiful yoga practice or time spent in nature. The mind rests in a tranquil state of awareness when the doshas are stable and balanced. This harmonious state, our essence nature, is what we seek to maintain as we move through life.

Rajas is the energy of action. It's stimulating and provokes movement, often leading to excess. It's also the energy that drives change, innovation, inspiration, and passion. Because rajas drives motion through action, it can create disequilibrium and imbalance. Too much rajas and we burn ourselves out, but not enough and we stagnate or feel stuck. When rajas dominates our mind with desire, our actions are often driven by discontent and anxiety.

Tamas is inertia. It is the energy of rest. It refers to stagnation, ignorance, heaviness, and attachment. Tamas has a dulling or slowing quality, often provoked from a lack of appropriate rajas. When tamas dominates our mind, we lack clarity and linger in indecision and inaction. Tamas can help calm or pacify us when we're overstimulated, but too much tamas can lead to depression, loss of desire, complacency, and laziness.

Just as the five elements shape your body and the world around you, all three gunas are necessary principles of creation. One is not necessarily better than another. You need rajas to move from tamas to sattva, and you need tamas to calm rajas and return to sattva. In simpler terms, you might need fiery activities in order to get off the couch and out of avoidant patterns. And other times, you might need to lie down, rest, and be still to calm overstimulation. But generally, our aim is to move toward sattva in our efforts. We want to use our awareness of how we're feeling in the present moment to observe when we're either too active or too stagnant and how our current state of mind influences our well-being. We can apply this awareness to our yoga practice, our relationships and work, what food selections we make, and all our decisions we're faced with each day.

Self-Inquiry

Can you observe how these different states drive your thoughts and actions? Do you tend toward one or another in your daily habits? Recall a time you experienced sattva. How did it feel in your body and mind?

Bridging Our Inner & Outer Worlds

We've explored the elements and doshas that make up the physical body, we've discussed the mind, now what about our senses? Our senses are the gateway between the outer world and our inner world. You know that saying, "If a tree falls in the forest, and there's nobody around to hear, does it make a sound?" This points to our connection between the mind, body, and senses. Our minds perceive an experience through the senses, our body reacts to it. Sensory input and our perception literally shape our entire world.

So, if nature speaks to us in her own language, it's one that replaces words with sensory experiences. The five sense organs—eyes, ears, nose, tongue, and skin—are bridges between the outer world and our inner realm. We communicate through our sensory organs and organs of action (*indriyas*) and make sense of the world around us through our mind (*manas*). Remember, each organ and action is connected to one of the five elements; in space, vibration brings sound to the ears; in air, movement brings touch to the skin; fire illuminates light to the eyes; through water, moisture brings taste to the tongue; earth brings smell to the nose. Based on these sensations and the memory of past experiences stored in it, the mind continuously generates thoughts and feelings, which in turn influence our actions.

Why are the senses so important to understand? Because knowledge is power, as they say. This cycle of perceiving and reacting is what shapes our entire perception of our reality. Most of the time we operate with very little awareness that this process is even happening! When I work with clients, our very first exercises are around developing an awareness of their senses, because it takes them out of the automation of action—that is, habit. We develop habits based on memory, and sometimes those habits serve us (like not putting your hand on a hot stove to avoid burning yourself), but often they leave us in patterns that aren't necessarily healthy. When trying to get out of unhealthy patterns of eating, binge-watching TV, or staying in painful emotional cycles, becoming aware of how sensory input influences us is key. My teacher has a saying, "How do you get out of jail? You have to first recognize you're in jail."

We're often blind to our patterns. Meditating on our senses and the intentional withdrawal of them is a way to get out of the habituated mind and into a real experience of the present moment. Our awareness and connection to all five senses is what informs the brilliant dialogue between our body, mind, and nature. When we develop this awareness through daily practice, we become fluent in identifying and nurturing our moment-to-moment needs. When we try new things, we break our habits—that is, we break out of jail.

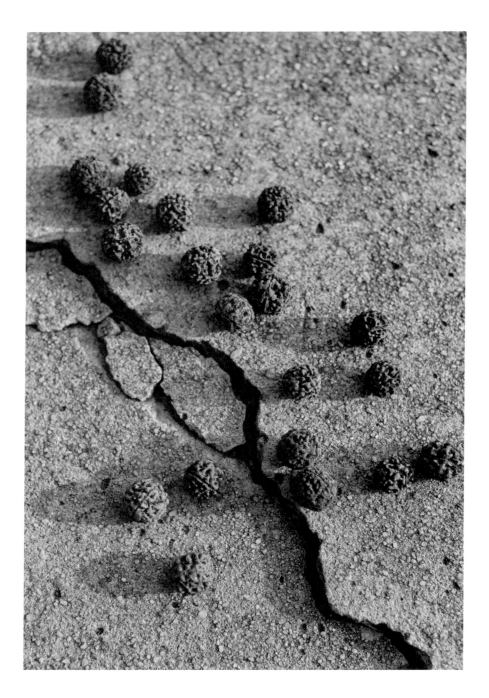

Learning to live each and every moment in concert with
the cyclical rhythms of the universe provides a solid
foundation for building a rich and wholesome life.

—BRI MAYA TIWARI

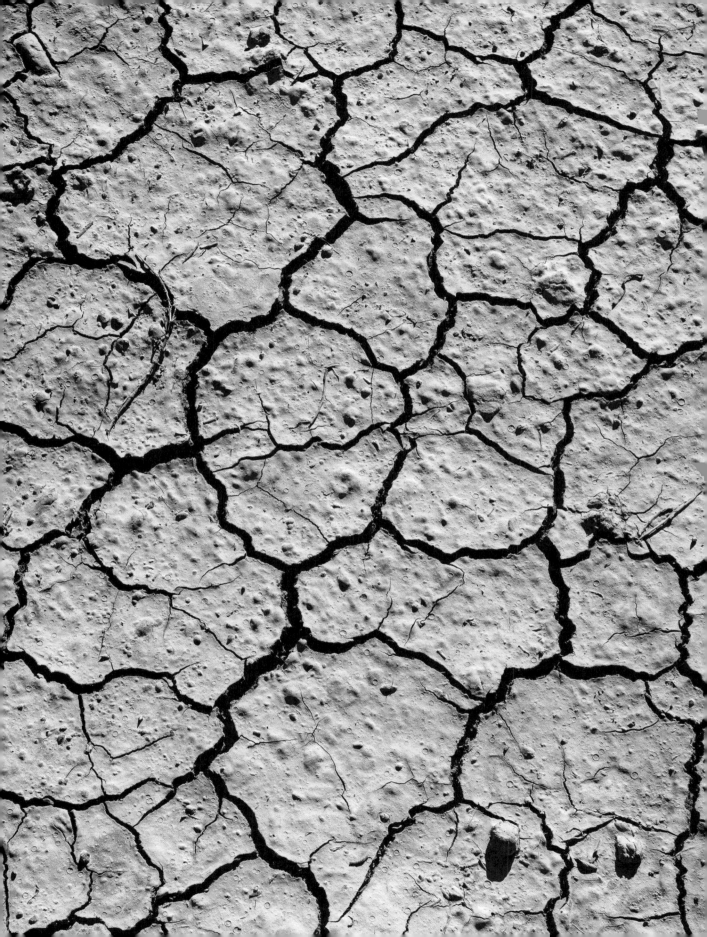

Self-Inquiry

Asatmendriyartha samyoga is the term that describes the misuse of our sense organs. Think scrolling through social media before bed and then having difficulty falling asleep. Or regularly smoking and eating really salty and spicy foods as a result of dull taste buds. There are many unconscious habits we have that lead to a different pathway of choice when our senses our overstimulated. Jot down a few ways you have misused your senses. What were the resulting actions?

THE ROLE OF TASTE

Food plays a crucial role in our health. The sense of taste does a lot more than inform satisfaction to our brain. Our tongue has the ability to identify how different foods will affect our body as well as our state of mind. Ayurveda classifies six primary tastes (*rasas*) within food—sweet, salty, sour, pungent, bitter, and astringent—each one connected to the five elements. These tastes can be discovered by mouthfeel. Like a skilled sommelier who can hold a sip of wine and note the subtleties of sweetness from berries or astringency from tannins in the vintage, a trained tongue can discern whether a food will move you toward balance or away from it. When we know that sweet foods contain the earth element, we understand it will have a grounding and nourishing effect that reduces vata—think roasted root vegetables in winter. Because sweet also contains the water element, it has a cooling and soothing effect that reduces pitta—think juicy watermelon in the middle of summer. When you start to learn the six tastes, planning what to eat becomes an intuitive process and can be used to balance your body through the seasons. This chart describes each taste, its associated elements and corresponding foods, and whether it will increase (↑) or decrease (↓) a particular dosha.

FOOD & CONSCIOUSNESS

Just as the six tastes influence the doshas, they can also influence the mind. Food, and how it is digested, has a direct effect on our consciousness. Sour, salty, and pungent foods contain the fire element; here, too much heat can lead to a rajasic mind. These foods include onions, garlic, fried and fermented foods, hot sauces, vinegars, and alcohol. A diet with too much of these foods can increase heat and lead to anger, agitation, a sharp tongue, an overactive mind, the inability to sit still or be alone, and frequent wake-ups throughout the night with racing thoughts or violent dreams.

The sweet taste has a pacifying effect, which can calm an overactive mind. But the quality of sweet matters. Processed sugar, ice cream and other frozen desserts, homogenized dairy, meat, oils, and wheat are all sweet in taste but create a sticky

THE SIX TASTES

TASTE	ELEMENTS	ACTIONS	EFFECT	FOODS
Sweet	Earth + Water	Builds tissues, calms nerves, relieves hunger	↓ Vata ↓ Pitta ↑ Kapha	Fresh and dried fruit, sweet vegetables (cucumbers, root vegetables, gourds), whole grains, natural sweeteners (honey, maple syrup, jaggery, coconut sugar), dates, fresh milk, and ghee
Sour	Fire + Earth	Lubricates tissues, stimulates digestion and elimination	↓ Vata ↑ Pitta ↑ Kapha	Unripe fruits, tamarind, lemons, limes, fermented and pickled foods (yogurt, kimchi, pickles, soy sauce, tamari, vinegars [ume plum, red, white], balsamic, apple cider)
Salty	Fire + Water	Increases flavor, absorption, water retention; hydrates colon	↓ Vata ↑ Pitta ↑ Kapha	Mineral salts, sea vegetables (kombu, nori, arame, wakame), water-based vegetables (celery, tomatoes, zucchini, cucumbers)
Pungent	Fire + Air	Increases heat; stimulates digestion and metabolism	↑ Vata ↑ Pitta ↓ Kapha	Hot and spicy peppers, black peppercorn, onion, garlic, ginger, mustard, horseradish, raw radishes and turnips, asafetida, cloves
Bitter	Air + Ether	Detoxifies and lightens tissues	↑ Vata ↓ Pitta ↓ Kapha	Aloe vera, dandelion, leafy greens, bitter melon, burdock root, eggplant, Jerusalem artichokes, sesame seeds and oil, dark chocolate, coffee, fenugreek
Astringent	Air + Earth	Absorbs water, dries and tightens tissues	↑ Vata ↓ Pitta ↓ Kapha	Legumes, raw cruciferous vegetables (cabbage, broccoli, cauliflower), fruits (pomegranates, unripe bananas, cranberries), basil, bay leaf, caraway, coriander, dill, fennel, marjoram, nutmeg, oregano, parsley, poppy seeds, rosemary, saffron, turmeric, vanilla, tannins in coffee, tea, and wine

Self-Inquiry

Take a look in your fridge. What foods do you gravitate toward? When you get a craving, do you crave sweets? Do you love salty and crunchy foods? Does every meal come with a hearty dose of sriracha on top? Our mental state usually drives our food choices. So, if you're feeling hotheaded and agitated, put away the hot sauce and ditch the coffee, and see how this can calm your mind as result. If you're reaching for the chocolate and baked goods night after night, ask yourself where you can bring more sweetness into your life through meaningful connections with friends and loved ones. Our craving for sweet often comes from a need for loving touch, kind actions, and connection. What are your cravings telling you?

and heavy quality that increases tamas. These heavy substances can slow us down and leave our mind dull when overconsumed. But when the sweet taste is consumed mindfully, it can have a sattvic effect that provides nourishment and contentedness. Choosing sweet vegetables, fresh fruits, quality organic dairy, and whole grains can help nourish a state of balance between the rajasic and tamasic effects of food.

No food is necessarily bad. It's all an experience of mind and body. But knowing what kind of experience will result from consuming different kinds of substances is what helps us make more conscious choices around how we nourish ourselves. We need all six tastes in our cooking to nourish the five elements and balance the doshas. In appropriate amounts, the six tastes can be used medicinally. In each seasonal section of the book, you'll find kitchen guides that outline what tastes and foods to favor or reduce in each season. We'll also explore more about the different tastes and how to work with them in a concept I like to call "the balanced bowl," which we'll discuss in the next chapter.

INTEGRATING THE SOUL

Life can be hard to navigate when we don't understand our greater role in the universe. Without a clear view or a path to guide us there, we might find ourselves grasping onto identities and false stories about who we think we are. This causes suffering and leads us away from svastha. True liberation and inner peace comes from knowing that beyond our physical form, we are limitless, we are the divine itself. These concepts can be hard to grasp when they are just that—concepts or words in a book. The aim of yoga and meditation is to help codify this understanding through our own direct experience.

Ayurveda recognizes six main philosophies that describe the origin and makeup of the material world and our relationship to it. These philosophies each present a viewpoint of reality that looks at the self as a part of the divine. There are many spiritual paths that are aimed to guide you toward this kind of mental liberation. In essence, there are many vehicles, but one path. Finding a well-practiced spiritual teacher can help you clarify your vehicle on the path. This is easily an entire book, or volumes of books, in itself! No matter your religious background, a great starting place is to simply sit in silent stillness for a few minutes a day. This spaciousness can invite your own contemplation and connection to the cosmic consciousness that Ayurveda describes.

BALANCING THE BODY & MIND

Now that you know the language of the elements, the doshas, and the gunas, you can start to identify imbalances as they arise. When a dosha accumulates over time, this longer term imbalance can lead to degeneration or disease. What causes the body and mind to become imbalanced? Life, and especially life at the fast pace we live today. Changes of environment, whether the natural shifting of the seasons or long-distance travel; changes to our routine; improper diet; stress; and overstimulation of our senses can all affect the balance of the doshas.

Signs of Imbalance

The best thing you can do is to be aware of the signs of imbalance and nurture your inner equilibrium with the appropriate diet and lifestyle practices.

While exploring these signs and symptoms of imbalance, keep in mind that you might experience some or all of these at different times of the year and seasons of life. Doshas naturally fluctuate due to seasonal influences, time of day, and stages of life. And the influences of modern life—disconnection from nature, processed foods and poor eating habits, travel across time zones, increased stress—especially contribute to dosha imbalance. Knowing what dosha imbalance looks and feels like in your body and mind can inform our daily choices that bring us back into balance instead of down a deeper path of disease.

The good news is that the doshas respond quickly to our food, lifestyle choices, and our thoughts! Once you recognize an imbalance, you make choices that stabilize the unstable dosha. To treat imbalance, Ayurveda often uses opposite qualities to reduce and support the elevated dosha or guna. Remember, *like increases like* and *opposites decrease each other*. In some ways, it's a cause-effect approach. You are cold, you drink cold water, you become colder. Or you are cold, you drink warm water, you become warmer. While this is a very simple example, it can be this intuitive.

By paying attention each day to signs of imbalance, you can make simple choices that encourage balance in your body and mind.

For example, I know that my vata constitution tends to make me more sensitive to cold, dry weather and seasonal transitions. Travel will also impede my digestion and make it difficult for me to stay asleep. To stay in balance, I maintain my daily routine while on the road, and always bring a bottle of sesame oil to do a grounding warm oil massage. I also rub oil into the bottoms of my feet before bed to help me sleep. In autumn and winter, I skip salads and eat more root vegetables and warming stews with a little extra ghee to keep me well-oiled and hydrated. On days when I feel overstimulated, my yoga practice includes longer rests and steady breathing to sooth my nervous system. I might even take a day or two with minimal talking and social media scrolling to give my mind a break and rebuild my energy reserves. Though these might seem like simple actions, I'm always amazed how quickly they bring me back into a balanced, sattvic state.

As you explore this concept of balance and imbalance, I want to share a word of caution to all my perfectionist friends out there. Balance is not static. It's not something that is ever fully achieved then sustained. In fact, the word *dosha* actually means "that which is quick to go out of balance" or "that which is at fault." Doshas very nature is to change. So, achieving a state of perpetual balance is not the primary goal of this system. Rather, it's about being in a state of observation and awareness. As you get to know yourself through this lens of the doshas, be gentle with yourself

	VATA	PITTA	KAPHA
IMBALANCED	Dry skin, hair, and nails Constipation, bloating, gas, and burping Popping joints, cold hands and feet Shifting pain in the body Tight, constricted, shallow breathing	Critical, sharp, angry, controlling behavior Overheating, excess sweating Red eyes, rashes, fever blisters Loose stools, acid indigestion Inflammation	Dullness, lethargy, greed, attachment, depression Weight gain, water retention, swelling, stagnation Excess mucous, sinus and lung congestion Sticky stools, slow digestion and metabolism
BALANCED	Clear, calm mind Free-flowing ideas and creativity Regular elimination and appetite Well-lubricated and freely moving joints Good circulation in hands and feet Free-flowing, easeful breath	Lightheartedness, good humor, humility, leadership Sharp thinking and comprehension, healthy discernment Steady appetite and metabolism Clear eyes and vision Rosy but cool complexion	Compassion, caring, kindness, devotion Strong immune system Vibrant eyes, skin, and hair Steady mind and motivation

along the way and approach your practice without judgment. Every day is a new opportunity to be a curious observer.

Nurturing Your Inner Fire

When I speak of our inner fire, I am speaking of *agni*—our essential digestive fire that governs the transformation of everything we take in through our senses. Agni's role is to transform energy into matter, whether this is turning nutrients into healthy tissue or food into consciousness. All roads lead back to digestion as the driver of good health. Ayurveda recognizes thirteen main types of agni within the body that help process and digest what we take in. In this book, what we're primarily paying attention to is our digestive capacity in our stomach and small intestines (*jathar-agni*), the main organs of digestion that transform the food we eat and turn it into the tissues that form our physical bodies.

Think of your belly's digestive fire as a wood-burning stove. It takes just the right amount of kindling, a few well-placed logs, enough space and a little air to stoke a hearty fire. Once the fire is burning, you want to feed it the right amount of fuel. If you stack too many logs on at once or not enough as it burns, you will put the fire out. Equally, if you throw a big bucket of ice water on top, you will douse the flames. Establishing a consistent routine around eating is like sustaining a good fire—you feed the flames just the right amount of food at the right time, giving space between meals to consume what was taken in before adding more. When running smoothly, a healthy digestion produces strength and vitality, but when affected, it can weaken, overheat, or dampen the inner fire.

SAMA AGNI (BALANCED AGNI)

Sama agni is the state of agni we strive to maintain for a steady and stable digestive fire. Sama agni can digest a reasonable quantity of any food in any season without challenge, keeping absorption and elimination in regular balance. Being "regular" may be different from your normal. In Ayurveda, healthy elimination is defined as an easy, well-formed bowel movement that occurs one to two times a day naturally without strain or stimulation by medications.

VISHAMA AGNI (VATA—VARIABLE/WEAK)

Vishama agni is associated with excess vata. This type of digestive imbalance causes an irregular appetite, variable digestion, abdominal distension, burping, gas, gurgling intestines, constipation (or alternating constipation and diarrhea), and colicky pain. Emotionally, it tends to cause anxiety, fear, and insecurity. Establishing a consistent eating routine of warm, well-cooked, and soupy foods can help to balance this type of digestive fire. Regular sleep and routines that create a sense of safety and stability in your life are also key.

TIKSHNA AGNI (PITTA—HYPERMETABOLISM/HOT)

Tikshna agni is associated with excess pitta. Pitta's light, hot, sharp, spreading, and subtle qualities normally support agni, but in excess they can inflame it—triggering overactive hypermetabolism and fast-moving elimination. Tikshna agni's strong fire creates an insatiable appetite for large quantities of food and the inability to skip meals without negative physical and mental consequences. Hyperacidity, acid indigestion, gastritis, heartburn, diarrhea, loose stools, ulcerative colitis, and other inflammatory conditions are associated with imbalanced pitta in the digestion. For this agni imbalance, limiting excessively oily, spicy, and inflammatory foods such as coffee, alcohol, and fried foods will help reduce internal heat. Soothing breathing and movement practices are also supportive. Laughter and humility can also go a long way to lighten up the excess in an overheated mind.

MANDA AGNI (KAPHA—HYPOMETABOLISM/SLOW)

Manda agni is associated with excess kapha, which dulls the appetite, slows the metabolism, and creates an experience of overall heaviness. Because of the cold, heavy, and dull qualities of kapha, a dull digestive fire can lead to regular colds and congested sinuses, lungs, and lymph. It can also contribute to weight gain and obesity, diabetes, hypothyroidism, hypertension, and hyperglycemia. A weak and dull agni can leave you feeling lethargic and sluggish. To balance manda agni, regular exercise and movement between meals can help metabolize and move the stagnant lymph. It's crucial to eat foods that are light, warming, and well spiced; fast until true hunger arises; and avoid snacking or grazing between meals.

HEALTHY ELIMINATION

Let's talk about bowel movements. We can eat all the healthy food in the world, but if we're not eliminating properly, we will encounter health challenges. Our bodies produce natural waste products (*malas*)—sweat, urine, and feces. When we're not eliminating these properly, toxins (*ama*) begin to accumulate and can lead to disease. Thus a healthy diet also requires us to pay attention to our elimination. Dry stools mean dry colon and high vata. Loose stools mean heat in the colon from high pitta. And sticky stools mean too much kapha. In your daily routine, observing your elimination patterns can help inform what diet choices to make that day to bring you back into balance.

EVERYDAY TIPS FOR HEALTHY DIGESTION

In the following chapters, you will find tips for tending your inner fire through the seasons. However, there are general guidelines that are great year-round and for all constitutions. If you're struggling to get your digestion on track, try integrating these practices into your daily routine:

- Establish a regular meal routine and stick to it. Avoid skipping meals and snacking or grazing all day. Space meals out by 4–5 hours to give time to digest and rest before eating again.

- Eat your largest meal at noon, when your digestive fire is highest.

- Opt for a simple cooked meal when your digestive fire is low. Raw foods, like salads, actually take more digestive capacity than a simple soup.

- Don't gulp liquids while eating, instead, sip warm water throughout the day to stay hydrated and wait an hour after eating to drink again. Skip the icy drinks and other cold beverages that douse your digestive fire.

- Only eat when you're truly hungry and when you're relaxed. Never eat when you're emotional or upset.

- Make eating the main event. Try eating in silence without conversation, technology or other distractions. When ready to eat, take 5 deep breaths to prepare your body to receive food. You can even say a small prayer of gratitude before your first bite.

- Chew your food fully to the consistency of a liquid before swallowing.

- If you've overeaten, lie or recline on left side for 10 minutes after a meal.

- Never repress an urge for elimination.

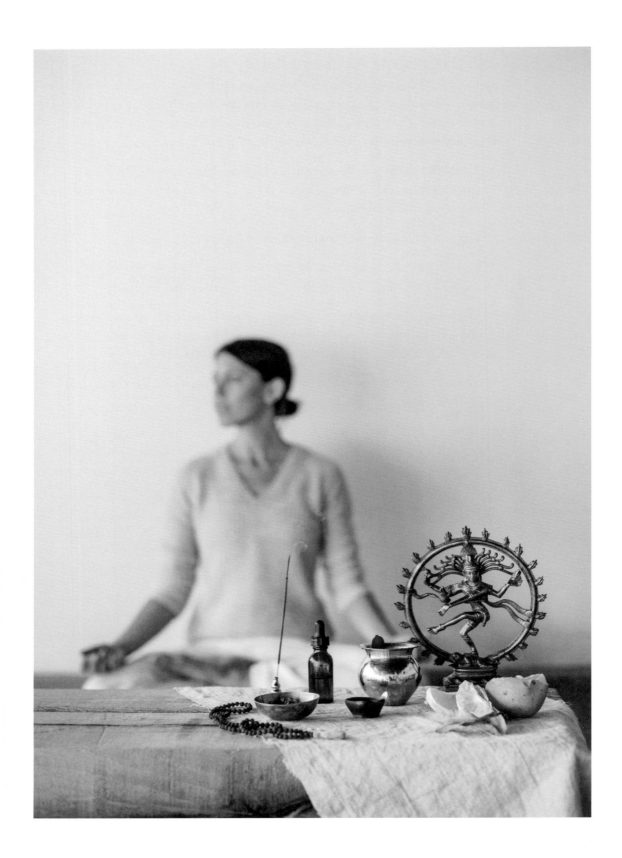

SEASONAL, LUNAR & DAILY CYCLES

Nature has rhythms and cycles influenced by the earth, sun, moon, and stars. These laws of nature impact our own internal rhythms. In our modern world today, we need extra support in this regard. Stimulated by artificial light, electronic devices, and almost instant access to anything and everything we desire, urban living has nearly disconnected us from our innate wisdom of nature. We're a culture that has forgotten how to eat, sleep, move, and live our lives in healthful and regenerative ways. The wisdom of an Ayurvedic lifestyle teaches us how to work with the intelligence of nature's seasonal, lunar, and daily rhythms—a theme you'll see throughout this book.

The distinct rhythms and cycles of our everyday lives also translates to the breadth of our life. If we divide an average lifespan into three stages of youth, middle age, and old age, one dosha will predominate in each stage. From birth into our youth, kapha governs this time of life. We have extra ojas, the subtle essence of a healthy kapha, that provides more juiciness and resilience to our bodies and minds. As we move into adulthood, pitta governs this middle-aged time of life where we have focused careers, family life, and greater responsibilities that require drive and focus. And as we age and slowly burn up our vitality, our bones become brittle, our skin dries, and our memory decreases; thus old age is characterized as a vata time.

Self-Inquiry

What rituals do you already practice in your life? How does this connect you to time and place?

Seasonal Cycles

Ritucharya, meaning "seasonal movement," describes the cycle of the seasons and the practices that connect us to them. It also refers to the timing of menstruation and conception. Each season expresses characteristics of a specific dosha. The ancient Ayurvedic texts describe six seasons, instead of the typical four we know with winter and summer divided into wet and dry months. This book is based on the Western four-season model of spring, summer, fall, and winter. Though the seasons greatly depend on our geographical location and its weather patterns, the general concept of balancing health through seasonal alignment is applicable to all. It's this seasonal awareness that allows us to live in greater harmony with our environment and the cosmic rhythms of the earth, sun, and moon and understand their effects on our biorhythms.

Lunar Cycles

The moon plays a significant role in our lives—influencing everything from our sleep cycles, energy levels, and moods, to the reproductive cycle and endocrine system of women. In nature, we see the influence on the ocean's tides and the ways indigenous farming practices used knowledge of the lunar cycles to plant and harvest crops. A lunar cycle is 29.5 days long and is divided into four primary stages: new, waxing, full, and waning. In the waxing moon, kapha is rising and peaks at the full moon. In the waning moon, vata is increasing and peaks at the new moon. Understanding the lunar cycles helps us understand and manage our energy accordingly. In part three, you'll learn about each lunar phase and how to work with the energy with different lunar rituals and reflective questions. Ladies, this is a particularly important cycle to observe! I've included a special section in each chapter for you to understand your own feminine rhythms and your powerful connection to the moon.

Daily Cycles

Dinacharya refers to our daily routine. In Sanskrit, *dina* means "day," "sun," or "flow"; and *charya* means "practice" or "conduct." This is perhaps the most important tool in a home practice and our connection to vikriti, because it helps us make informed decisions around what foods to eat and yoga practices to do to bring the doshas into balance each day. Dinacharya particularly emphasizes morning as our most sacred time, as these hours create the foundation for the rest of the day and help clear wastes (*malas*) to bring us back to a neutral state before the start of the day. However, this routine encompasses the full arc of a day, breathing mindfulness into each moment from the time you wake up to when you sleep. In the overstimulated world we live in, a daily routine provides a helpful outline for keeping us on track with the rhythms of the day. I'll outline the routine and practices in detail in "A Recipe for a Daily Practice" in part two.

The Ayurvedic Lifestyle Clock

You've probably heard of circadian rhythms before. Circadian science, or chronobiology, is the modern science that supports the ancient wisdom of Ayurveda's seasonal and daily routines. Circadian science details when certain physiological processes happen in relationship to darkness and light, based on roughly the twenty-four-hour time clock. The Ayurvedic lifestyle clock shows how our own biorhythms relate to the cycle of the sun and moon throughout the day, the lunar month, and the year. With this knowledge of time (*kala*) we learn how to sleep, eat, breathe, and move in alignment with the macrocosm. And when we live and flow in this harmony, we're more likely to stay in balance over the course of the year.

The inner circle of the chart shows the division of the three doshas in relation to the hours of the clock, moving from daytime to nighttime. The middle displays the corresponding gunas that describe qualities of the doshas, while the outer circle shows how the doshas correspond with the seasonal influences. Since this book is already structured to explore the four seasons with recipes, rituals, and practices to support the related dosha, this section will look more closely at how the doshas influence us throughout the course of a day.

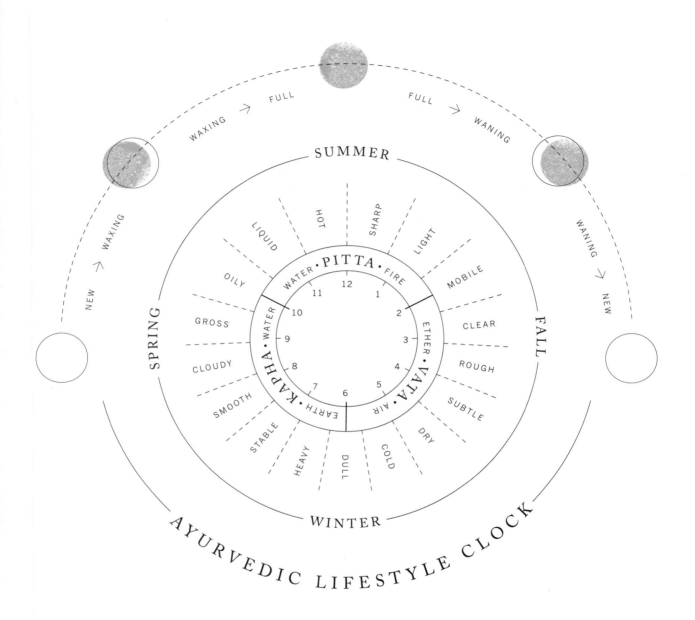

6 A.M.–10 A.M. / 6 P.M.–10 P.M.

Kapha dominates these morning and evening hours. An increase of water and earth elements in these hours can bring slow digestion, increased mucus, and a feeling of heaviness, especially if we eat late and then sleep in late. Waking up with or before the sun will ensure we feel light and ready to greet the day. Equally, eating lighter at night than you have earlier in the day and getting to bed before 10 p.m. can ensure better rest and an easier time falling asleep.

10 A.M.–2 P.M. / 10 P.M.–2 A.M.

These are peak pitta hours. Daytime is when the sun and our inner fire are at their peaks. The daytime pitta hours are optimal for scheduling meetings, getting the bulk of our brain work done, and eating our largest meal—around noon, when digestive fire is strongest. The nighttime pitta hours explain why we can get a second wind after 10 p.m. and stay up late with more energy. But working late at night ends up depleting us in the long run. It's better to get to bed before we start to burn the midnight oil too many nights in a row.

2 A.M.–6 A.M. / 2 P.M.–6 P.M.

Vata governs these early morning and late afternoon hours. With the air and space elements dominant, it's a great time to be creative, vision, and dream. Vata brings a sense of lightness and mental clarity in the morning hours, making before the sun rises the easiest time to meditate and practice yoga. In the late afternoon, we often feel fatigued from the day's stimulation and reach for a nervous system stimulant, such as coffee or chocolate, to keep us going. This is an ideal time to take a short nap or practice restorative meditation, such as yoga nidra. The Spanish have siesta, or an afternoon rest, as a cultural practice for a reason!

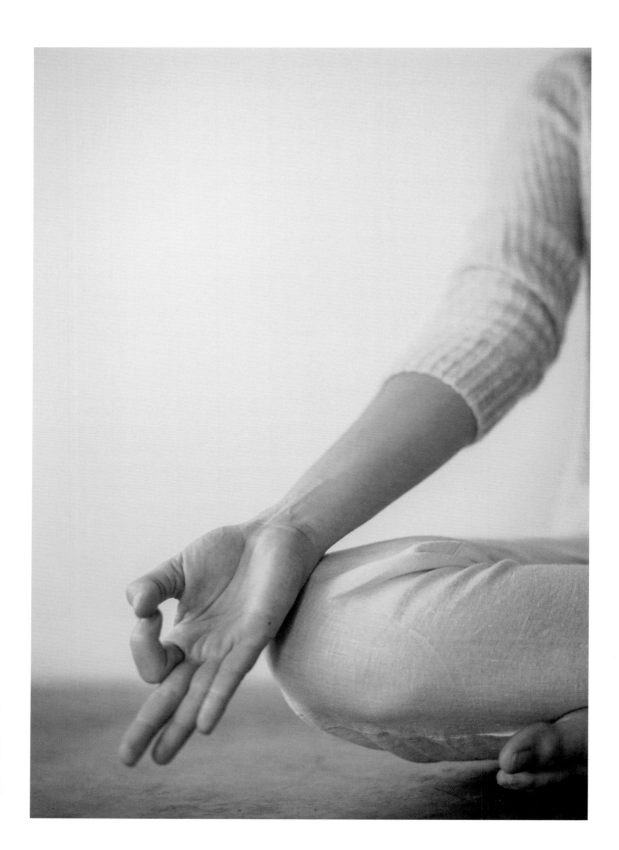

THE AYURVEDA &
YOGA CONNECTION

Yoga is considered to be Ayurveda's sister science, with a similar timeline of development. Many know yoga in the modern West as a physical practice, a workout for staying in shape. However, until recently, yoga was primarily a practice for spiritual liberation, only outlining a handful of postures for meditation. It wasn't until the early 1900s that yoga became a more embodied practice and started to merge with Ayurveda as a means of supporting the body, mind, and spirit as an interconnected whole.

Yoga can be used as a therapy (*cikitsa*) to prevent and treat disease. Because the mind influences the body, yoga's aim is not only to bring strength and vitality back to the physical body but also to restore the mind back to its sattvic state so that it can perceive reality more clearly. What you'll find in this book is an outline for how to use the physical postures (*asana*) and breathing practices (*pranayama*) therapeutically to balance your body and mind throughout the seasons.

What Are Asana and Pranayama?

Asana is the collective name for physical postures used in yoga. *Asana* can also be used to describe the movement in and out of a posture. There are standing, seated, and prostrate postures that include various twists, folds, backbends, and lateral movements. The aim is to provide strength, stamina, and suppleness to the physical body and mind in preparation for meditation. Movement into each posture is paired with the breath. An asana is mastered when it becomes steady and effortless; we are relaxed and at ease in each pose and each breath. Marrying movement and breath in specific sequences is known as *vinyasa*. While asana can be considered exercise, it's also a therapy and a contemplative practice that gifts you greater self-knowledge.

In this book you'll also find breathing practices for each season. These breathing practices are called *pranayama*. *Prana* means "vital energy," and *ayama* means "to expand or extend." In practicing pranayama, we aim to cultivate and expand our vital energy by altering the flow of our breath and focusing our mind. There are five types of prana connected to the doshas that describe the movement of prana in the body—inward (*prana*), downward (*apana*), upward (*udana*), horizontal (*samana*), and outward (*vyana*). Patanjali's *Yoga Sutras* (1.31) observes how disturbances of our body and mind can alter our breathing patterns. Conversely, our breath has the power to influence our mind and balance our body. When we are aware of the different ways prana moves, we can use specific pranayama practices to balance the doshas and cultivate greater vitality. Because pranayama can be quite powerful, it's helpful to work with a trained teacher to learn more about the subtleties and ways to work with prana in a purposeful way.

Working with Yoga through an Ayurvedic Lens

Yoga as a therapy is not a one-size-fits-all or all-the-time approach. Rather, yoga can be practiced in accordance with your unique type (prakriti) and day-to-day needs (vikriti). There is a diverse array of options available today in the modern yoga industry; my aim with this book is to equip you with an understanding of how you can use yoga as a therapeutic tool to balance the doshas and experience firsthand how different postures and breath influence your body and mind.

VATA-BALANCING YOGA

To balance the light, mobile, and erratic nature of vata, your yoga practice should be steady and stabilizing. Sequences should emphasize grounding, warming, increasing circulation, and a downward movement of energy (*apana vayu*). Because erratic, tight, and shallow breathing can occur when vata increases, your yoga practice should emphasize long and full inhalations to circulate prana and provide a sense of nourishment. Slow, rhythmic, and repetitive sequences connected with your breath satisfy the need for movement but in a stabilized container. Standing poses should focus on connecting to the earth through your feet and hugging muscles to the bone to protect your joints. A steady, focused gaze maintains attention and counters a wandering mind. Seated postures, such as forward folds and hip openers, draw energy to your pelvis and calm your nervous system. A long Savasana and Yoga Nidra meditation with blankets to keep your body warm and your joints supported are invaluable for restoring a frazzled body and mind. When vata is elevated, it's essential to create a consistent daily practice routine, even if just for 10 minutes.

Consistency and routine are great allies when overwhelmed with change. You can find the vata-focused asana and pranayama sequences in the Fall and Winter chapters.

PITTA-BALANCING YOGA

To balance the hot, sharp, and intense qualities of pitta, your yoga practice should be cooling, quiet, and noncompetitive. Avoid hot yoga, fast-paced classes with loud music, or practicing in front of mirrors where self-criticism and competition can arise. A practice that encourages surrender, compassion, humility, and acceptance can soothe an overactive pitta. Keep your gaze soft and focus attention inward. To release built-up heat, your breathing should emphasize long exhalations and slow, rhythmic, gentle ujjayi breathing. Sequences should be active enough to satisfy the desire for movement, but never too much that it becomes overheating or aggravating. Moon salutations, or sun salutations practiced without intensity, are an example of this. Twists, seated forward folds, and restorative inversions (legs against the wall) are all beneficial. When overheated, do not cover your body with a blanket in Savasana. Switch up your daily routine and avoid getting too rigid or attached to doing the same thing every day. Explore the pitta-focused asana and pranayama sequences in the Summer chapter.

KAPHA-BALANCING YOGA

To balance the slow, dense, and heavy qualities of kapha, your yoga practice should be vigorous, energizing, and uplifting. Building heat through sun salutations, longer holds in standing postures, and more active ujjayi breathing is key. Emphasize diaphragmatic breathing to bring more air into your lungs. Because kapha's primary seat is in the heart and chest, poses such as backbends that move energy upward and break up stagnation are helpful. Inversions such as Downward-Facing Dog, Shoulderstand, and Headstand relieve water retention and increase circulation. Chanting mantra and kirtan or listening to uplifting music can bring a lightness and devotional quality that balances kapha. Prioritize a morning yoga practice to keep the energy flowing. Find a kapha-balancing sequence in the Spring section.

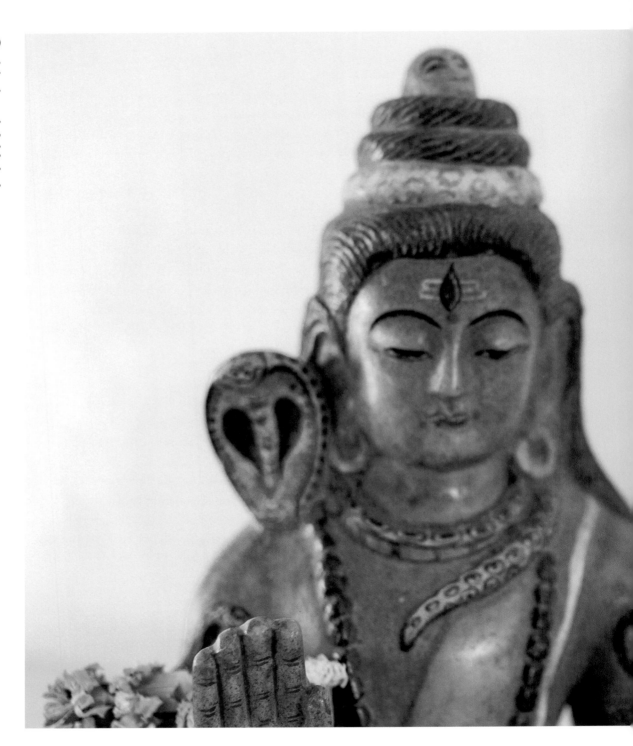

PART TWO

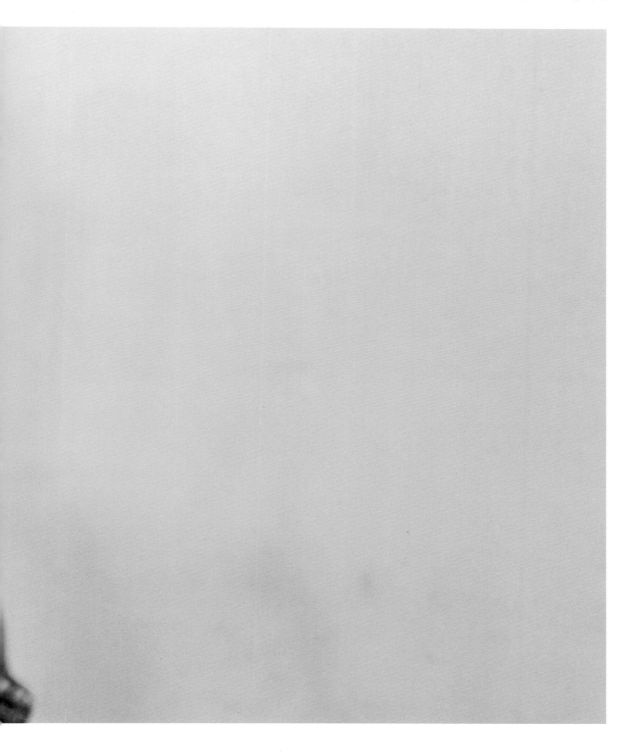

PREPARING FOR

YOUR YEAR

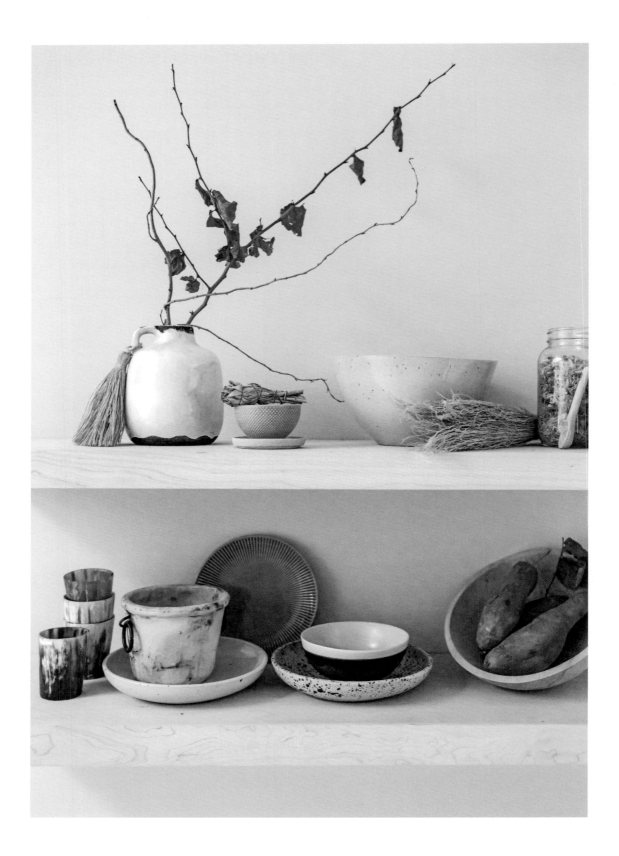

HOW TO USE THIS BOOK

This book is your companion to living a vibrantly rich and well-nourished life. Guiding you through an arc of a year, you'll learn you how to stay in harmony with the different cycles of the day, the moon, and the seasons. Within each seasonal chapter, you'll explore different yoga practices, rituals, and recipes that support the dominant dosha of the season. Spring focuses on balancing kapha, Summer focuses on soothing pitta, and the Fall and Winter sections explore ways to nourish vata. No matter our prakriti, our personal constitution, we are all affected by seasonal transitions. And no matter our climate, we are influenced by these passages of time throughout the year. The aim is to practice paying attention to your environment and how you're feeling each day.

We are each unique, with bodies that have their own stories to tell. The wisdom of Ayurveda teaches us that no single practice fits everyone all the time. With this in mind, you'll find "Dosha Notes" in the seasonal recipes and yoga sequences to give you ideas of how to modify for the different doshas as needed to meet your needs. For example, if you are experiencing a pitta imbalance, you'd follow the modifications for pitta in the yoga practices and recipes.

Some recipes are nourishing for all three doshas, and in this case there will not be modifications noted. If you're unsure what modifications to make, refer back to the Self-Inquiry practice on page 12.

Symbols	Ⓥ = Vata	Ⓟ = Pitta	Ⓚ = Kapha

The Practices

Each season incorporates asana and pranayama for the different doshas. The sequences in this book are simple but powerful. And in a world of so much stimulation, *less is more*. By slowing down and practicing simply but consistently, you'll begin to create a relationship with these practices and experience how they nourish you in different times of need.

You can approach these practices as physical exercise, or you can view them as sadhana, a spiritual practice. As my teacher reminds me, anything can be done with a devotional heart and mind. I invite you to approach everything in this book—from the time you step onto your mat to the moments spent preparing food in your kitchen and everything in between—as an opportunity to practice loving presence.

As you explore these yoga sequences, view this time as a sacred space to get to know yourself through a new lens. Notice how the postures affect your mind. Notice how intentional breathing influences your energy. Practicing yoga has the power to increase our awareness of our inner rhythms and patterns and put us back in touch with the guidance of our inner teacher.

When you wake up each morning and do your self-inquiry practice, you may note that you need more intensity and vigor on the mat to move you out of stagnation. Or perhaps you are feeling anxious and overwhelmed, so you take a more calming approach with longer rests. The yoga sequences in each section are designed to balance kapha in spring, pitta in summer, and vata in fall and winter, respectively. However, the way you approach these sequences can also be adapted to balance the doshas as needed for your body type and daily needs.

PRACTICE PROPS

I recommend the following props for your home practice space:

- Yoga mat
- Cork blocks
- Strap
- Bolster

- Yoga blankets
- Meditation cushion
- Folding chair
- Eye pillow or cloth to cover the eyes

A Note of Caution: Please use your discernment when practicing yoga at home. If you have injuries, if you are recovering from illness or surgery, or if you are pregnant, it's especially recommended to consult your doctor and work with a certified practitioner to help you craft a personalized yoga and lifestyle plan. This book is not meant to diagnose, treat, or prescribe based on your personal constitution or imbalance.

BREATH & MOVEMENT

Ujjayi is a breathing technique used while performing the yoga postures. It is done entirely through the nose while keeping the mouth and jaw relaxed. It is a diaphragmatic breath, meaning your rib cage should expand fully when you inhale and contract when you exhale. This deeper breathing pattern allows more oxygen into the body and produces an energizing but balancing effect. This breath has an audible "HA" sound to it, the same sound if you were to breathe heavily against a mirror to fog it up. Try this: Take a deep breath in, open your mouth, and pretend you're breathing out against the glass. Do this again, but close your mouth as you exhale and make the "HA" sound. This is ujjayi breathing. It is synchronized with your movements to help build internal heat while you move. It can be practiced more forcefully to increase heat and circulation, or more gently in times when you're overheated. The main aim is to remain aware of how you're breathing while practicing the yoga sequences.

ALIGNMENT

Sthira-sukham asanam in the *Yoga Sutras* describes how each posture should be approached with steadiness and ease. Yes, we want to pay attention to our physical alignment; how our knees are bent at 90 degrees over our ankles in lunging postures; how engaging our pelvic floor muscles and transverse abdominis can stabilize our pelvis and support our spine; how our index fingers face forward and our hands are firmly rooted on the floor when bearing weight in postures such as Downward-Facing Dog. All of these guidelines are important, and working with a practitioner can help you identify the subtleties of alignment. But what's most important in your home practice is your awareness of your inner alignment—how you're approaching and arriving into each posture as a way to direct prana. Ayurvedic doctor and author Dr. Robert Svoboda reminds us that cultivating steadiness (*sthira*) and ease (*sukha*) as we move through the days and seasons of our lives establishes a foundation for fully realizing our spiritual aspirations, accomplishing our worldly goals, and weathering the inevitable changes and difficulties that come our way. The aim of practicing yoga is not to perfect the shapes of the poses but to cultivate prana, tejas, ojas, and a greater awareness of our true nature.

The Rituals

Life can pass you by quickly, especially in the busy, hyperconnected, and overstimulated world we live in. The saying "How you do anything is how you do everything" means that you have a choice to live mindlessly or with awareness. For me, seasonal and lunar junctures offer a time for reflection. They help me take stock of where I spent my energy and make conscious choices about where I want to direct my focus in the cycle ahead. The rituals included in this book offer ways to create a meaningful pause from your day-to-day routine and infuse intention into your life. Whether it's gathering friends together for a joyous summer solstice celebration outside or invoking our inner fire with a fire ceremony on the new moon, these moments help us feel more connected to the cycles of the earth, sun, and moon, creating a different relationship to time in the process. In each section, you'll learn about the energies of the four phases of the seasons and the moon with rituals that connect you to them.

Tip: At the start of the year, go through your calendar and mark the days of the equinoxes and solstices. Look ahead at a lunar calendar and input all the full and new moon days into your monthly calendar. This helps me plan my social activities, travels, personal rituals, and rest days so I can use my energy and time more efficiently.

The Recipes

Conscious cooking is one of the quickest ways to balance the doshas and connect with nature. The simple, everyday recipes in this book highlight seasonal ingredients and tastes to nourish the doshas and support your digestion.

Food also tells a story. What you'll find in these recipes are stories of my relationship to food through my years of travel, studies, and creative explorations in the kitchen. You'll find influences of my Italian-Portuguese family lineage. You'll taste flavor combinations and cooking techniques I picked up from my Lebanese friends in college, my summer living in South India, and my time spent working in a commercial raw food kitchen. But above all, I designed these recipes with great care and attention to the specific ingredients.

This isn't your standard vegetarian cookbook. Each season's recipes use specific ingredients that highlight the six tastes and bring balance to the related dosha focus of the season. For example, the Green Tea Broth Bowl (page 123) is a light and refreshing springtime soup that uses astringent green tea, buckwheat soba noodles, and pungent ginger to support kapha. You won't find heavy grains or roasted root vegetables as the foundations of a spring recipe. Instead, you'll find lighter grains such as amaranth and millet, pops of vibrant sprouts, and fresh bitter greens that

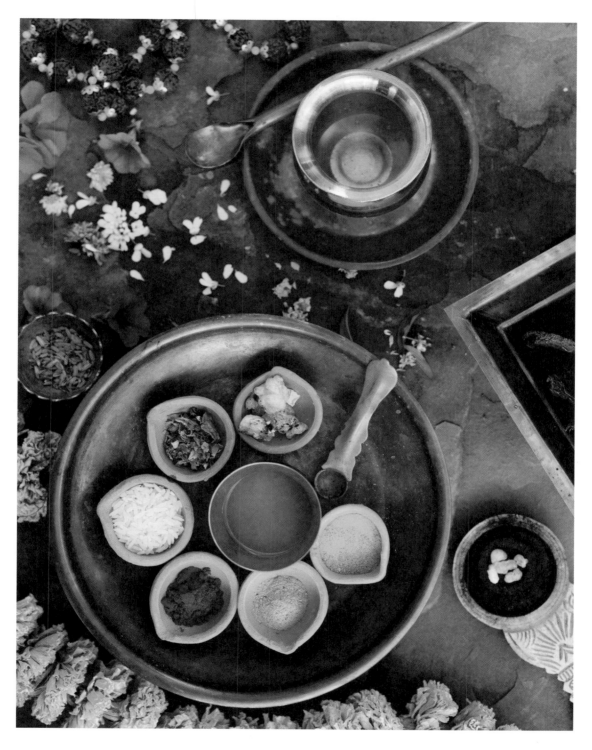

Sadhana is being present with everything we do.

—BRI MAYA TIWARI

support natural cleansing to help you lighten up. Summer's recipes emphasize sweet and cooling ingredients in the hot months. Fall focuses on grounding and building foods that are oily, soupy, and dense. And winter uses warming spices and healthy fats for extra nourishment in the colder months. As the weather can be fussy and so can your personal needs, don't hesitate from time to time to jump into the season that is present that day.

You'll also find lots of plants in this book. In fact, this whole book is based on a wholesome plant-centered diet of organic fruits, vegetables, nuts, seeds, grains, and legumes. There are accents of dairy, such as a yogurt dipping sauce or a sprinkling of goat cheese. But these are optional and can be enjoyed or skipped over. I also offer recommendations for nondairy alternatives.

While these recipes are primarily plant-centered, I do offer some ideas for how to mindfully consume animal products without aggravating the doshas. You'll also notice the occasional use of onions and garlic, which you don't typically find in books related to yoga. This is because traditional Ayurveda actually doesn't look at any one substance as bad, but rather encourages awareness of how it affects the body and the mind and using with intention. So, intentionally, you'll find a few pungent flavors in the cooler months where a little more heat can be helpful in your diet. If you find these too stimulating, there are modifications for that, too.

What you won't find are tons of expensive superfoods from distant places. The bulk of these recipes use simple, everyday ingredients. There are a few specialty spices you might need to order online. I've included my favorite places for ordering oils, herbs, and other unique ingredients in the resources section.

Lastly, you won't find any dietary dogma here. I don't label recipes as vegan, gluten-free, lectin-free, or any other exclusive titles. Rather, I emphasize cooking simply, cooking with loving awareness, and creating an experience that brings you joy in the kitchen and around the table. My hope is you get playful in the kitchen, connect with the sensual experience of cooking and eating, and have fun with it!

A NOTE ON DONENESS: COOKING WITH INTUITION

When I first started writing this book and set out to create the recipes, I quickly realized I never actually use measurements when I cook. In most of my early written recipes, the instructions would say something like "Remove from oven when done." In the recipe-testing process, much of the feedback I received from my testing group was "What does 'done' mean?"

So, how do we know when something is done? Cooking is truly an intuitive process more than a calculated one. Gained through a symphony of cues our senses have gathered over time and fine-tuned through experience, our intuition guides us on subtle levels—from how long to cook the food to the right amount of spices to perfectly flavor the dish. Conscious cooking isn't a fixed formula but rather a very personal art form. The way I like to use spices may not be the way that a dish calls to you.

My invitation to you here is to trust your intuition and tune in to your senses to guide you in the kitchen. Don't be afraid to mix and match, to try new things, or to put your own twist on a dish. You might burn or botch a few recipes along the way, I sure did more than a few times, but the end result is a greater confidence and wisdom on how to nourish yourself. And often, it's from that space of emptiness in our mind and full presence in our heart that guides us to create the most magical meal.

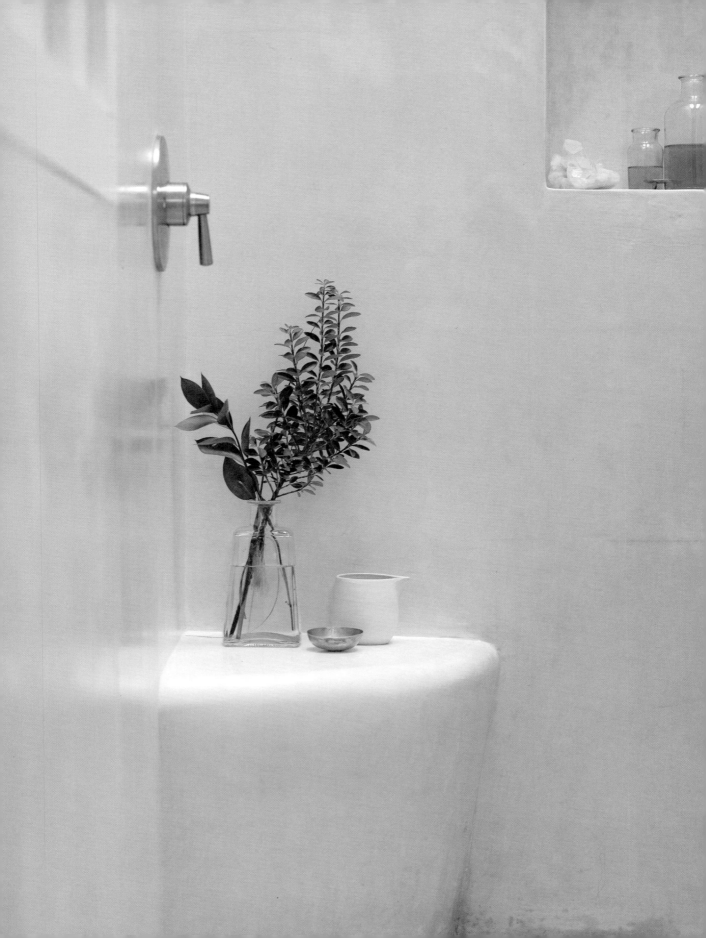

RECIPE FOR A DAILY PRACTICE

Setting the tone for your personal practice starts with creating a sacred space that you will nourish and, in turn, nourish you. *Saucha* is the yogic principle of cleanliness. This means tending the temple of your home and keeping your belongings tidy as a way to support a clutter-free mind. As you begin, start by organizing your home and turning it into a sanctuary you look forward to being in. Prioritize beautification in your kitchen and personal practice space, breathing life into these corners of your home that will hold you as you journey into self-exploration.

In your kitchen, rid your pantry and fridge of old foods and spices you haven't touched in years, stock and organize the shelves with wholesome ingredients that are easy to see and reach, and bring in fresh flowers or plants that breathe life into the space.

In your yoga practice space, set up a cozy area that feels inviting and safe. You'll need a yoga mat; yoga props such as a cushion, blanket, strap, and block; and a journal and pen. Build an altar on a low table that you greet each day. On your altar place sacred objects and pictures of teachers or those who inspire you, to help direct your attention toward where you're going and what you're focusing your energy toward. Include a scent-free candle or ghee lamp. Each morning, I like to light a candle as a way to purify and honor the space and welcome in a new day. Offering fresh-cut flowers and fruit on the altar is another beautiful way to nourish the intentions of your practice and give gratitude to your teachers.

However you choose to adorn your spaces, make sure you devote time to building these sacred places you'll return to each day. With an inviting space, you're more likely to step into new practices and cultivate healthy daily habits.

Dinacharya: Your Daily Routine

One of Ayurveda's most powerful tools is *dinacharya*, the outline for a daily self-care routine. This daily routine gives you tools for caring for your body and mind. It's also a practice of self-inquiry and an opportunity to observe what imbalances might be present that day. Your tongue, eyes, nose, skin, urine, bowels, and sweat can all tell you what doshas are elevated. Look back to page 22 for the characteristics of balanced and imbalanced vata, pitta, and kapha.

If you've had a variable schedule or no routine at all, this outline can take some time to get used to. I recommend picking one or two of these practices and committing to them for a month, or until they become a natural part of your rhythm. You might experience a learning curve when incorporating new practices into your routine, but eventually you'll nail your pacing and timing, and feel the tremendous benefits of the routine you can't live without!

SELF-CARE ESSENTIALS

- Natural-bristle dry skin brush or silk *garshana* gloves

- Organic plant oils

- Ceramic neti pot

- Nasya oil

- Eye-rinse cup

- Tongue scraper

WAKE UP

Waking with the sun is an essential part of a healthy lifestyle rhythm. This means getting to bed by 10 p.m. so you can wake by 6 a.m. or earlier. There are specific times that are best to wake for each constitution: vata, 6 a.m.; pitta, 5:30 a.m.; kapha, 4:30 a.m. For all, waking in the quiet predawn hours (*Brahmamuhurta*) is the most beneficial time for doing your meditation and yoga practice. This may take some time to get used to, but you'll notice big effects on your energy levels throughout the day following this waking-sleeping rhythm. As you wake up, take a few moments to set an intention or say your prayers. Keep your phone or computer out of the bedroom and wait until you've finished your morning routine before checking emails or watching the news.

ELIMINATE

Ideally, you want to have a bowel movement shortly after you wake up. But if you don't, the following practice will typically help you to go naturally. Reliance on coffee and other stimulants can aggravate vata and pitta over time. Instead,

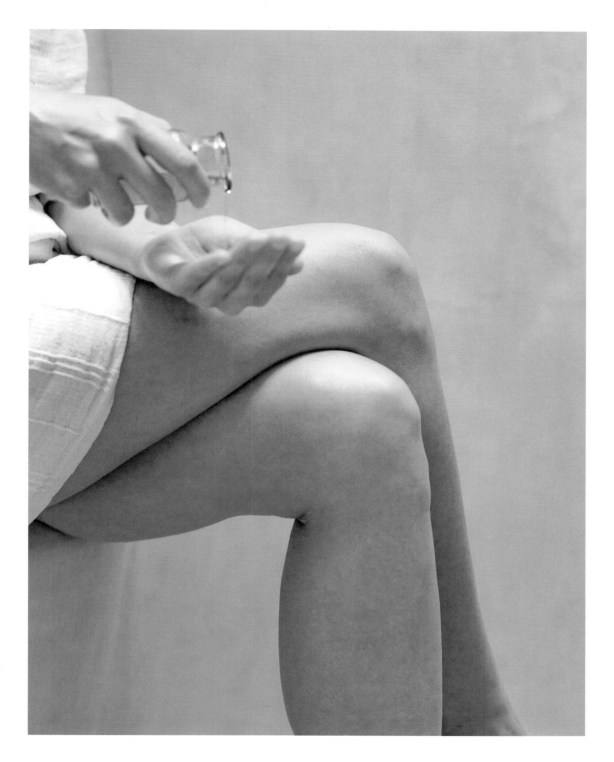

We benefit most from following the natural rhythms and cycles of nature and tuning ourselves to this, rather than creating our own artificial time.

—DR. VASANT LAD

try sipping warm water or doing gentle self-massage on your abdomen, twists, and deep, slow belly breathing to support daily elimination in your morning routine.

DAILY CHECK-IN

Malas are the waste products your body produces each day. Your urine, bowel, and sweat can tell you a good deal what doshas are elevated. As you move through your morning cleansing routine, notice the qualities of your morning eliminations and take a look at your skin, eyes, and tongue. Are they dry? Hard? Oily? Soft? Dull? Sharp? Hot? Cold? Look back at the twenty qualities and their opposite pairings; these will help you decide what food, movement, and self-care practices you'll need for your day.

CLEANSE YOUR EYES: EYE RINSING

Splash your face and open your eyes with cool water. Blink and look clockwise, then counterclockwise, with your eyes. If you have itchy, dry, or red eyes, an eye-rinse cup with cool water and a few drops of rose hydrosol (pure rose water, not essential oils or alcohol-based tinctures) can soothe irritated eyes.

CLEANSE YOUR MOUTH: OIL PULLING & TONGUE SCRAPING

Your mouth is the gateway to your digestive tract; cleansing it before eating or drinking is crucial. Oil pulling (*gandush*) is the first step to cleansing your mouth. This is the practice of swishing oil around your mouth to remove bacteria from your teeth and improve gum health. It also reduces vata. You can use coconut oil, untoasted sesame oil, or an herbal oil pulling formula. Take 1–2 tablespoons, and without swallowing or gargling, simply swish the oil around your mouth for 5–20 minutes. I will often multitask and do my oil pulling while I heat water for the kettle or do my dry brushing and shower. When done, spit the oil out in the trash can, and use a stainless steel or copper tongue scraper to gently scrape your tongue 5–7 strokes. Tongue scraping removes the excess bacteria and oil from the tongue. Finish your mouth-care routine with brushing your teeth.

CLEANSE YOUR NOSE: JALA NETI & NASYA

Jala neti is the practice of rinsing your nasal passages with purified water to clean your sinus cavities of excess mucus. Use a ceramic neti pot filled with warm water and about ¼–½ teaspoon of non-iodized salt. Over a sink, lean forward and tilt your head to one side so your ear faces down toward the sink. Place the spout to the nostril facing up and lift the pot so the water slowly drains into one nostril and out the other. Use half the pot on one side, then gently blow your nose to clear out mucus, and repeat on the other side to finish the pot. When you blow your nose, be sure to blow gently through both nostrils to protect your ears. Never forcibly blow your nose or plug one nostril; keep both open. Neti is particularly helpful in spring when congestion and seasonal allergies are high. Finish with tilting your head back and applying a few drops of nasya oil, an herbal nasal oil, or sesame oil into each nostril. Neti might not be in your everyday practice but rather a part of your weekly routine or your self-care tool kit when you have seasonal allergies or congestion, especially in springtime. Nasya can also be done on its own as a practice to lubricate your nasal passages and stimulate mental clarity. This is especially great in cold, dry months or climates, and when traveling.

CLEANSE YOUR SKIN & LYMPH: DRY BRUSHING

Dry brushing (*garshana*) uses a natural-bristle brush or raw silk glove to remove dead skin and stimulate lymphatic drainage. Start at your feet and work upward toward your heart, using gentle pressure and long strokes with repetition. Dry skin brushing is very stimulating, so this is one practice you'd definitely want to do in the morning instead of nighttime. This is a highly beneficial practice for reducing kapha, especially in springtime and late winter or when you experience water retention and weight gain. Skip dry skin brushing when vata is high, as it can be too aggravating; instead, focus on oil massage.

NOURISH YOUR TISSUES: ABHYANGA

Of all the practices, oil massage (*abhyanga*) might be the most important in a daily routine. It has the potential to support all three doshas, soothe the nervous system, calm inflammation, stimulate the lymph, and nourish all the tissue layers of the body. It's a powerful practice! This oil massage is best done before you shower or bathe. By bathing after, the warm water helps the oil penetrate deeper into the tissues while also protecting the skin's natural oils. For your oil massage, use an organic plant-based oil. For vata, try untoasted sesame oil, which is naturally heavy and warming; for pitta, try coconut oil, which is cooling and light; and for kapha, try apricot or almond oil, which are light and neutral. Herbal infused oils are also wonderful.

Warm the oil by pouring a few ounces into a small glass and placing it in a larger glass filled a quarter of the way with piping hot water. This acts as a double boiler to quickly warm the oil. Lay a towel on the floor or toilet, to sit on. Start from the crown of your head and rub both ears; work your way down to your feet. Use long strokes on the long bones and circles around the joints. Around your breasts, move in circles directed toward your heart, and use clockwise circles around your navel. Moving from your head down to your feet has a calming, supportive effect, especially for vata and pitta. To support kapha, you might start at your feet and move upwards to the head. A simple oil massage can be done as a short 5-minute session in the morning, or a longer 30- to 60-minute experience. The longer you massage, the deeper the oil penetrates the seven tissue layers. Think of this more as a nourishing therapy rather than just a moisturizing routine.

BATHE

Following dry skin brushing and oiling, finish your cleansing rituals with a shower or bath. Bathing is a form of meditation. A hot shower or bath not only helps induce a light sweat and open up the skin and sinuses but also remove past impurities you no longer want to hold on to as you start a fresh day.

HYDRATE

Sip a glass of hot water with a squeeze of lime or lemon juice to stimulate your digestion. If needed, have a small sip of water when you wake up, but enjoy the rest of your morning beverages after you've done your mouth-care routine.

ASANA, PRANAYAMA & MEDITATION

Once you've cleansed your sense organs and eliminated, begin your yoga practice. This can be done before or after bathing. This doesn't have to be a 2-hour endeavor; some mornings, this may be a few rounds of pranayama and a couple of sun salutations. The aim here is to cultivate prana not endure a rigorous workout. Try the seasonal sequences in each chapter's yoga section.

MEALS

Conscious eating is an important part of a daily routine. Establishing set mealtimes supports healthy digestion and elimination. It's best to eat breakfast before 8 a.m. or fast until true hunger arises at lunch. Don't skip lunch! Eat a satisfying lunch between 11 a.m. and 1 p.m., and a light dinner by 6 p.m. Maintaining a consistent eating schedule helps to stabilize blood sugars and avoid overeating after going too long without food. Planning your meals and prepping them ahead of time ensures that you'll stay with this recommended rhythm of eating.

REST

A short 10-minute nap or guided meditation, such as yoga nidra, can help replenish a tired body and mind in the afternoon. Rest when fatigued rather than pushing through with more caffeine or other stimulants.

WIND DOWN

Try an evening oil massage and hot bath to wind down, or simply rub oil into the bottoms of your feet before bed to calm and ground you. Turn off any electronics and read, journal, or meditate before bed. Creating a healthy evening routine is just as essential as your morning practices.

SLEEP

Sleep is the wet nurse of our health; it is crucial to aspects of our well-being. In the nighttime hours, our organs rest and regenerate, wastes are metabolized, and emotions are processed in our subconscious mind. Be in bed by or before 10 p.m. so you don't catch that second wind in the evening pitta hours.

Self-Inquiry

Prajnaparadha is the Ayurvedic term that describes when we know the outcome of an action but still do the thing that doesn't make us feel great. Think staying up late binge-watching a series on Netflix and eating ice cream. You know it'll lead to poor sleep and feeling heavy the next day, but you do it anyway. These "crimes against wisdom" repeated over time can lead to imbalance. Write down a few of your habits or obstacles that inhibit you from maintaining a healthy daily routine.

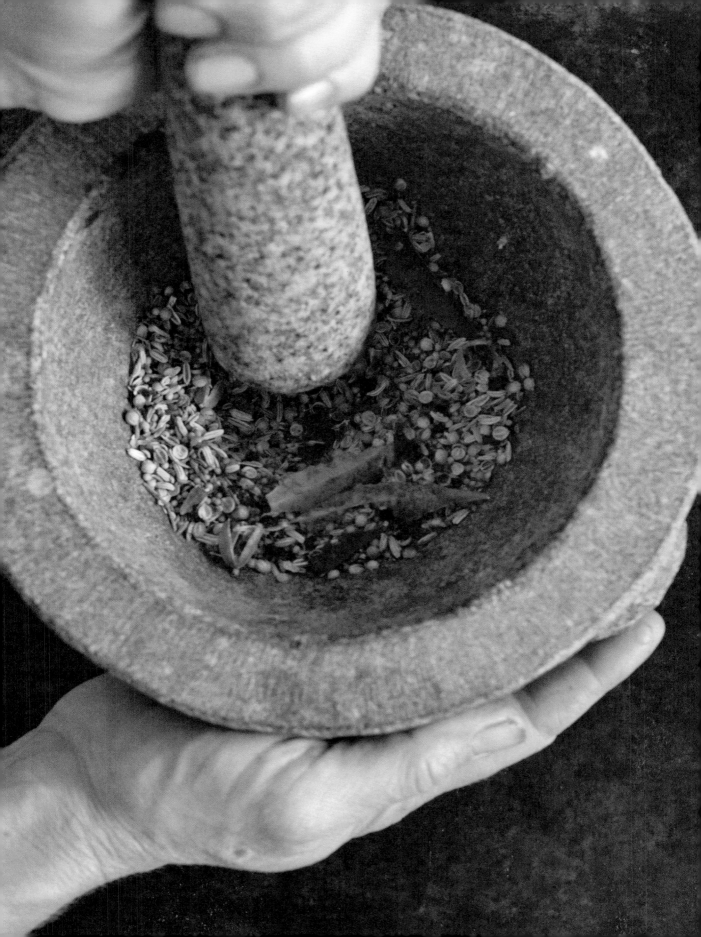

KITCHEN WISDOM

How do you eat well when you have a busy schedule? The simple answer: be prepared and organized. It makes all the difference to have the right tools and ingredients ready to use in your kitchen. Here, I share my favorite cooking tools, pantry essentials, and prep tips to set you up for a year of joyful home cooking.

Essential Equipment

Simple tools made from earthen materials, your hands, a present mind, and a loving heart are all you need to make a nourishing meal. When setting up your kitchen, there are a few staples you'll return to time and time again in your cooking endeavors. Note that most of the recipes you'll find in this book use basic cooking methods, though a few do call for a blender, food processor, or juicer. Rice cookers are also helpful. It's also best to avoid cookware that contains harmful chemicals, such as Teflon and aluminum. Instead, when shopping for kitchen equipment, look for items that use natural materials such as wood, clay, cast-iron, and steel. These are optional but helpful items in a modern kitchen.

- Ceramic and earthenware pots

- Cast-iron skillets

- Stainless steel saucepans and pots

- Pressure cooker

- Baking dishes, sheets, and pans

- High-speed blender

- Wooden utensils

- Quality knives

- Microplane or handheld grater

- Fine-mesh sieve or colander

- Cheesecloth or nut milk bag

- Spice grinder (mortar and pestle, *molcajete*, *suribachi*, or electric coffee grinder)

- Thermos (for taking food or hot beverages on the go)

Stocking Your Pantry

Ayurvedic cooking is often associated with Indian cuisine, with good reason. This wisdom comes from India and thus the food is influenced by the culture. However, Ayurvedic cooking doesn't limit you to one cuisine or cooking style. Rather, cooking Ayurvedically means to align with nature and use your understanding of the elements in the kitchen to create harmony in your body and mind through food. You select foods with qualities and tastes that balance your constitutional and seasonal needs while still celebrating your own cultural culinary traditions.

A traditional Ayurvedic diet does not rely heavily on the regular consumption of eggs, meat, or fish. Rather, these proteins are used with a medicinal intention to treat an imbalance or specific need. If you choose to eat animal products, seek out local small-scale farmers who have relationships with the animals and ethical farming practices. When we consume animal products, their lives become a part of ours. Take time to honor those lives in your kitchen preparations and eat with awareness.

In my pantry you'll find staple ingredients I keep stocked year-round. Many of these staples can be used in a dynamic number of ways depending on the cooking method and what other ingredients I pair them with. Instead of shopping for a single recipe, I buy my spices, grains, and legumes in bulk to stock my pantry. Here are some of the staples I recommend keeping in your kitchen.

GRAINS	OILS	SWEETENERS	VINEGARS	LEGUMES	NUTS & SEEDS
Amaranth	Coconut oil	Coconut sugar	Raw apple cider vinegar	Adzuki beans	Almonds
Barley	Ghee	Dates	Ume plum vinegar	French lentils	Chia seeds
Basmati rice	Olive oil	Jaggery		Red lentils	Hemp seeds
Brown rice	Sesame oil (untoasted)	Maple syrup		Split yellow mung dal	Pistachios
Buckwheat	Sunflower oil	Raw honey		Whole green mung beans	Pumpkin seeds
Millet					Sesame seeds
Oats					Shredded coconut
Quinoa					Sunflower seeds
					Walnuts

SPICES: STOCKING, STORING & GRINDING

Spices are an essential part of an Ayurvedic kitchen. Why? Because spices are an easy way to incorporate the six tastes into your meals and they can be used medicinally to balance the doshas through the seasons.

Stock your spice cabinet with whole seeds instead of ground spices. Often those little jars of ground spices you find at the grocery store are stale and may have been sitting on the shelf for years. If you have old spices in your pantry, compost them and start fresh. Food should be filled with prana and enhance your life force when you eat them. Whole spices retain oils better than pre-ground spices, and their potency is released when freshly ground. Buy a coffee grinder to grind your seeds into fine powder. A mortar and pestle (sometimes called a suribachi or molca-jete) is another way to grind spices by hand.

Store your spices in clear glass jars with labels that are easy to read. In India, a *masala dabba* is another way to store spices for quick use. These handy little stainless steel boxes come with a number of small cups inside for organizing spices. I like to grind my spices for the week and organize them in the masala dabba. Each season I reorganize my spice box to include the spices I'll use most for that season.

Cooling	Warming
Basil	Ajwain
Cardamom	Anise
Coriander	Allspice
Dill	Asafetida
Fennel	Black Peppercorns
Mint	
Flower waters	Chilies
Parsley	Cinnamon
Saffron	Clove
Tarragon	Cumin
Turmeric	Ginger
Vanilla	Mineral salt
	Mustard seed
	Nutmeg
	Pippali

Meal Planning

Ayurvedic wisdom promotes eating meals that are life-giving, fresh, and filled with prana. When you buy frozen premade meals to be reheated, you're consuming something with very little life force left in it. Equally, eating food several days after it's been cooked and sitting in the fridge will have a different effect on the body and mind than eating a meal freshly cooked that day. With a little planning and prepara-tion, eating well doesn't have to be taxing on your time.

PLANNING AHEAD

Lack of time is a common complaint to eating nourishing home-cooked meals. Planning meals for the week ahead can help cut down on the confusion of what to eat while saving time, money, and food waste along the way. I like to map out my menu by looking ahead at my workweek, social events, and seasonal needs. From there, I plan a few specific meals and write my shopping list to also include a few of my regular produce staples (think cilantro, leafy greens, root vegetables, and fresh dairy). This way I know what recipes I'm anchoring around while still having some flexibility to mix and match fresh ingredients in a quick meal or balanced bowl. I also keep a rotation of whole grains, legumes, nuts, and seeds soaking the night before I go to bed, making it easy to throw on a pot of quinoa and mung bean soup or a quick blend of fresh almond milk in the morning.

BATCH PREPPING

Instead of batch cooking, which makes you a big pot of something to reheat and eat throughout the week, I like batch prepping, so I can quickly and easily cook fresh meals each day with ready-to-use ingredients. After grocery shopping, I take time to wash, peel, and cut some of my more durable ingredients. This might mean cubing root vegetables and storing them in a container in the fridge for the week, so I can toss them in oil and roast them quickly for dinner. Or trimming and cutting leeks, scallions, shallots, or ginger to store in a jar for quick access. With lighter, more perishable ingredients such as greens, I may wash and cut these the night before use. I also prep jars of preblended spice mixes for making a chai, chutneys, kitchari, or other soups and stews.

COOKING FOR ONE, TWO, OR A FEW

As a rule of thumb, when cooking for one person, 2 hands cupped together is the desired portion for a meal that will satisfy your stomach's needs without overfilling it. This is about a ¼ cup of dried beans or rice and 1 handful of raw cut vegetables or 2 handfuls fresh cooked greens. With this in mind, you can scale back the recipes if you're cooking for one or double a recipe if you're cooking for a few. Generally, all the recipes in this book are made to serve 2–4 portions or people.

How to Build a Balanced Bowl

Ayurvedic cooking became enjoyable for me when I stopped getting hung up on the long lists of foods for the doshas and started understanding the more fundamental principles of foods themselves. Does a food build my body or lighten my body? I recommend revisiting the six tastes chart (page 19) to see how each taste comprises the elements. These six tastes can be divided very simply into two categories: building and lightening.

When looking at these two categories, you'll find building foods contain tastes that have more water and earth elements, which are grounding and nourishing; lightening foods contain more fire, air, and space elements, which have a cleansing or reducing effect.

BUILDING (SWEET, SOUR, SALTY)	LIGHTENING (PUNGENT, BITTER, ASTRINGENT)
Animal proteins	Legumes
Whole grains	Nuts
Fresh and cooked fruits	Seeds
Sweet vegetables	Raw vegetables
Dairy	Greens
Oils	Fresh herbs
Sweeteners	Spices

Generally, a meal should comprise about 60 percent building foods and 40 percent lightening foods. By doing so, we're simultaneously assisting both the nourishment and regeneration of the tissues. With too many building foods in a single meal—think the American staple diet of meat, potatoes, and buttered bread—we feel full and heavy, which can weaken our digestive fire. With too many lightening or cleansing foods, we are never fully satiated and tend to swing the pendulum to snacking on sweets and salty foods for balance. This is why eating solely green salads never really works for sustainable weight loss or a satisfying life. But if you were to add some cooked quinoa, roasted vegetables, a handful of seeds, and a creamy tahini dressing, your green salad would become a balanced bowl. When I learned how to use these principles of combining intentional foods and flavors, it took the confusion out of what to cook and eat each day, and made creating nourishing meals fun, easy, and attainable.

My desire is that each recipe in this book inspires your own creative exploration in the kitchen. Don't get stifled by the "rules" or let self-doubt come in the way of trusting your own inner wisdom. Rather, trust your senses to guide you in mixing and matching different recipe components to meet your palate and build a balanced bowl. With this concept, you can deconstruct and adapt the seasonal recipes to create an endless combination of flavorful new dishes to satisfy your daily needs and desires. The beauty of the balanced bowl is that it gives me freedom and flexibility to adapt to the dynamic environment around me while satisfying my taste buds and honoring my body's needs each day.

How to Build a Balanced Bowl

Grain
(30%)

+

Sweet
Vegetable
(30%)

+

Legume
(20%)

+

Bitter
Vegetable
(20%)

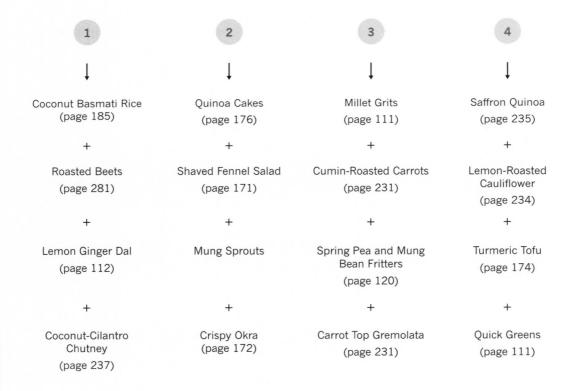

1

↓

Coconut Basmati Rice
(page 185)

+

Roasted Beets
(page 281)

+

Lemon Ginger Dal
(page 112)

+

Coconut-Cilantro
Chutney
(page 237)

2

↓

Quinoa Cakes
(page 176)

+

Shaved Fennel Salad
(page 171)

+

Mung Sprouts

+

Crispy Okra
(page 172)

3

↓

Millet Grits
(page 111)

+

Cumin-Roasted Carrots
(page 231)

+

Spring Pea and Mung
Bean Fritters
(page 120)

+

Carrot Top Gremolata
(page 231)

4

↓

Saffron Quinoa
(page 235)

+

Lemon-Roasted
Cauliflower
(page 234)

+

Turmeric Tofu
(page 174)

+

Quick Greens
(page 111)

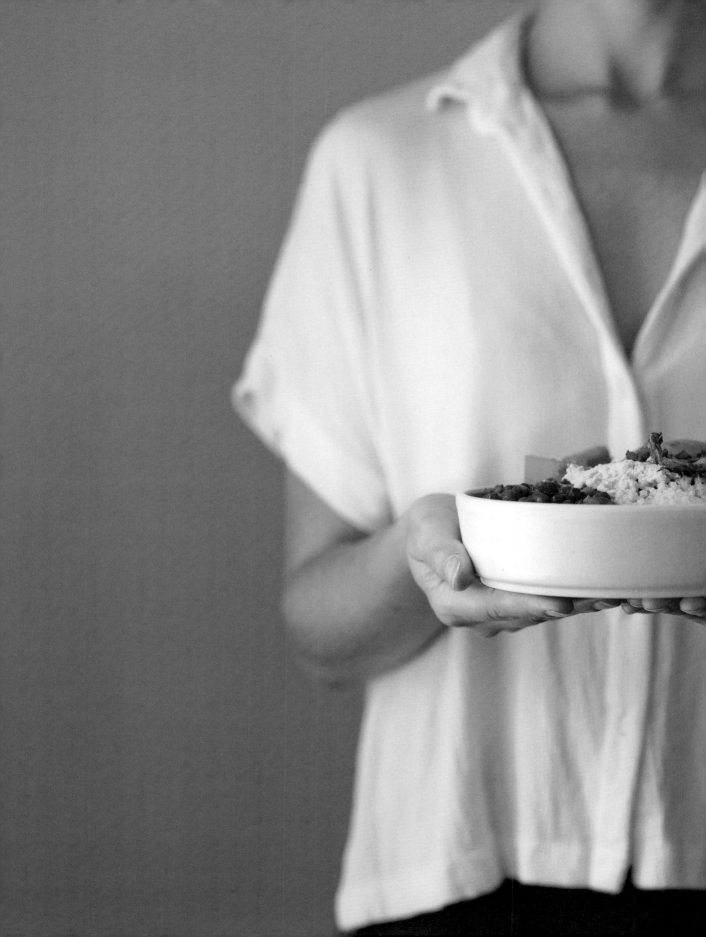

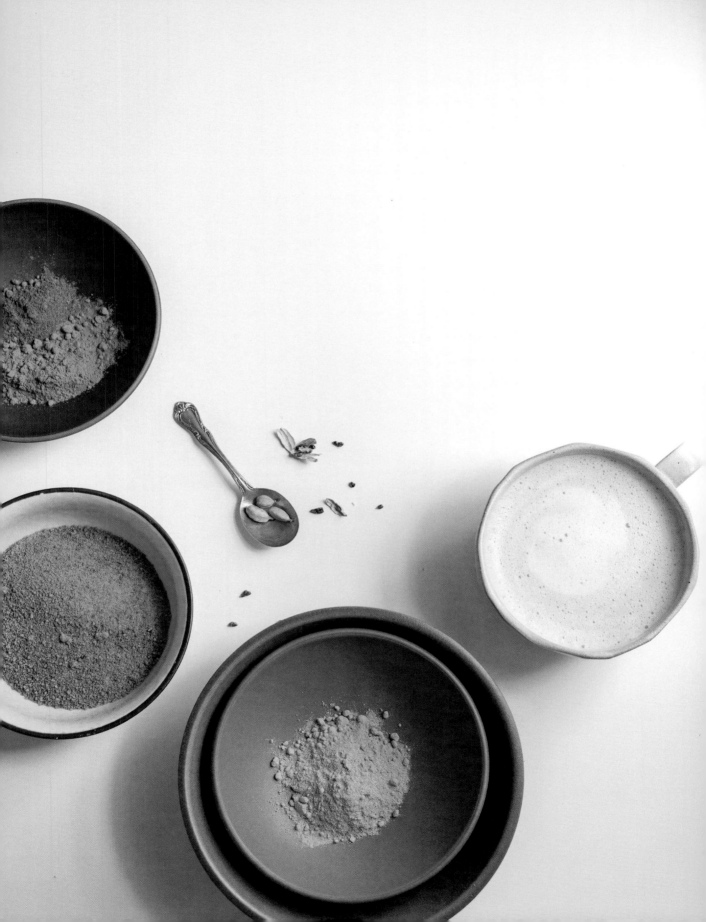

All-Season Recipe Staples

Ginger Appetizer

This quick recipe makes a great appetizer to kindle digestive fire before a meal. The sour and pungent tastes of fresh ginger and citrus awakens the taste buds and get digestive juices flowing. Serve on spoons to your guests before sitting down for dinner. Additionally, if you wake feeling full or have scanty appetite or indigestion, this is a simple trick to help support digestion.

PREP: 2 minutes | YIELD: 1 serving

¼ teaspoon grated or finely minced fresh ginger

Pinch of Himalayan pink salt

Squeeze of lime or lemon juice

Place the ginger on a spoon and sprinkle with a pinch of mineral-rich salt and a bit of lime juice. To eat, chew slowly to release the juices.

Instant Chai Powder

This instant chai powder is my travel go-to. Add it to hot water or stir it into steamed milk for an easy herbal tea that boosts digestion with its blend of warming spices. This mix is also wonderful in morning porridge—try adding it into breakfast kanji or oatmeal.

PREP: 5 minutes | YIELD: 12–24 servings

½ cup coconut sugar or jaggery

2 tablespoons ground ginger

2 tablespoons ground cinnamon

1 tablespoon ground cardamom

1 teaspoon ground nutmeg

¼ teaspoon ground cloves

Combine all ingredients in a bowl and stir to blend. Transfer to a clean, dry jar and seal with a lid. Store until ready to use. This blend will last 1–2 months in a sealed jar stored out of direct sunlight. When using, add 1–2 teaspoons of chai powder to 1 cup of hot milk or water.

CCF Tea

CCF (Cumin Coriander Fennel) Tea is a tridoshic tea, meaning it's good for all body types and all seasons. Cumin's slight astringency and pungency balances vata and kapha, while fennel and coriander calm pitta. Together, they relieve bloating and reduce indigestion. Make a hot pot in the morning and store in a thermos, so you can sip slowly throughout the day between meals for digestive support. The savory tea might be a new flavor experience at first, but it will quickly become a favorite once you experience the benefits!

PREP: 2 minutes | COOK: 10 minutes | YIELD: 4 servings

4 cups water

1 tablespoon cumin seeds

1 tablespoon coriander seeds

1 tablespoon fennel seeds

In a small pot, bring water to a boil and add the spices. Simmer for 5 minutes. Turn off the heat and steep for another 5 minutes before straining. Store in a thermos or jar, sip warm between meals. This tea is best brewed fresh and enjoyed warm each day.

Digestive Lassi

Just as the name states, this traditional Ayurvedic drink is best consumed at the end of a meal to aid digestion. For a sweet variation, try cardamom in place of cumin. While fruit sounds tempting, keep it simple with spices alone to avoid difficult-to-digest food combinations.

PREP: 2 minutes | COOK: 1 minute | YIELD: 1 serving

¼ cup fresh plain yogurt

½ teaspoon finely minced or grated fresh ginger

¼ teaspoon ground cumin

½ cup warm water

In a blender, combine the yogurt, fresh ginger, ground cumin, and water. Blend until creamy. Pour into a glass and sip slowly at room temperature.

Ghee

Ghee is a staple in an Ayurvedic lifestyle, from cooking to self-care remedies and rituals. Similar to clarified butter in the culinary world, ghee is made by slow cooking unsalted butter to separate out the milk solids. The result is an easy-to-digest, versatile cooking oil. Ghee cooks well at high temperatures, making it a great alternative to more delicate oils when sautéing or roasting vegetables. You'll also find ghee used in skin-care and eye treatments, for medicinal herbal remedies to help deliver the nutrients deeper into the body's tissues, and even in ceremonial candles to burn at an altar.

PREP: 5 minutes | COOK: 30–45 minutes (15 minutes per 1 pound of ghee) | YIELD: About 2 cups

2 pounds organic, high-quality unsalted butter

In a heavy-bottomed saucepan, melt the butter on medium heat. Reduce heat to low and cook for 20–30 minutes, allowing a thick foam to bubble up to the top of the pan. This foam is both water and milk solids evaporating. Most of the foam will begin to cook out, but occasionally you can skim the excess foam off the top and discard. A traditional practice is to chant mantras over the pot while you skim, infusing this golden nectar with the loving energy of the mantra. Even listening to mantra music while you cook can change the energetic resonance of the food.

Continue this process of skimming and gently stirring clockwise every few minutes until the foam is boiled off and the bubbling has stopped. Look for a golden-hued translucent liquid. Ghee can quickly go from perfectly done to burned, so keep the heat low and keep an eye on the butter. If you have a very hot stovetop, you may position the pot slightly off the flame to avoid cooking too quickly.

Note: Make sure your utensils and jars are completely dry before using; water in the containers can contaminate the ghee. And be sure to use a clean utensil each time you dip into the jar to avoid bacteria that could cause it to mold or spoil. Resist the urge to lick the ghee spoon and double-dip!

Once done, remove from heat and allow to cool for 15–20 minutes. Slowly strain the ghee through a fine-mesh strainer covered with a paper towel or several layers of cheesecloth, into a clean, dry jar. Allow to sit on the counter uncovered for another 15 minutes to continue cooling before sealing with the lid. Place the sealed jar in the fridge to set. You can store at room temperature for up to 1 month, or longer in the fridge. If you live in a humid climate, consider storing in the fridge to avoid molding, and pull it out to soften just before cooking.

Nut & Seed Butters

I love using nut and seed butters for everything from frothy lattes and truffles to creamy dressings and sauces. But many store-bought nut butters are frequently rancid and some even include added preservatives and processed sugar. Homemade nut and seed butters are easier to make than you think. Keep a few varieties of nuts and seeds stocked in your pantry for a rotation of fresh butters ready to use.

PREP: 5 minutes | COOK: 10 minutes | YIELD: 2 cups

2 cups raw, unsalted nuts or seeds (almonds, walnuts, pecans, cashews, macadamias, pistachios, Brazil nuts, sunflower seeds, sesame seeds)

¼ cup sunflower or untoasted sesame oil

Place the nuts or seeds in a food processor and grind 2–3 minutes, until you have a coarse powder. Stop and scrape down the sides. Continue grinding until the course powder starts to turn into a paste. Repeat scraping the sides periodically to incorporate evenly into the mixture. If the mixture gets too hot, stop to let it cool down for a few minutes. If the mixture feels dry, especially for something such as sesame seeds, you can add a bit of untoasted sesame oil to the mixture if you're making tahini, or sunflower oil for other seed and nut butters. Store in the fridge for up to 4 weeks.

FLAVOR VARIATIONS

| TO SWEETEN | 2–3 tablespoons raw honey or maple syrup |
| | 2–3 tablespoons coconut sugar or jaggery |

TO SPICE	1 tablespoon vanilla extract
	2 teaspoons ground cinnamon
	1 teaspoon ground cardamom
	½ teaspoon dried ginger

Mantra Milk

When the mundane becomes the sacred, we experience the beauty of each small task at hand. This recipe for almond milk gets the name "Mantra Milk" from the somewhat meticulous process of peeling the skins of soaked almonds by hand. With each almond you can recite your mantra or affirmation, turning a seemingly mundane task into a meaningful meditation. Swap or add in cashews, hazelnuts, hemp seeds, or sunflower seeds to make a variety of delicious nut and seed milks. Try steel-cut oats or basmati rice soaked overnight for a whole grain option. For a thicker creamer-like consistency, reduce ratio to 1 cup nuts to 2 cups water. For other flavor ideas, try seasonal variations below. These homemade milks will last 3–4 days in the fridge and taste vastly better than anything you can buy in a box!

PREP: 8–12 hours for soaking | COOK: 5–10 minutes for peeling and blending | YIELD: 4 servings

1 cup raw almonds

4 cups filtered water

Pinch of salt

Optional: 2 tablespoons maple syrup, raw honey, or 2 pitted Medjool dates, to sweeten

Place the almonds in a medium bowl and cover with filtered water. Soak overnight, until skins start to separate from the nuts. Remove the skins by rubbing each nut between your fingers, placing the peeled almonds in a new bowl and discarding the skins.

After the almonds are peeled, rinse and drain again. Transfer to a blender and add the filtered water, salt, and the sweetener or spices here, if using a seasonal variation. Blend until smooth and frothy. Pour through a nut milk bag, cheesecloth, or other fine-mesh strainer to separate the pulp from the liquid. Store the milk in an airtight container in your fridge.

Note: Soaking almonds removes an enzyme inhibitor known as phytic acid from the nut and makes it more digestible. Peeling the almonds makes a creamier almond milk and reduces the drying and heating qualities the skins have. But if in a time crunch, you can make almond milk without removing the skins. Simply rinse and drain after soaking, then transfer to the blender.

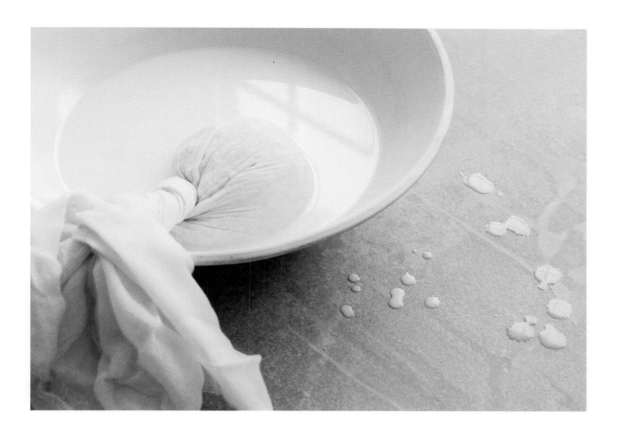

SEASONAL VARIATIONS

STRAWBERRY CARDAMOM MILK (SPRING/SUMMER)	10–12 fresh strawberries, stems removed 1 teaspoon ground cardamom 1 tablespoon raw honey Pinch of salt
COOLING COCONUT ALMOND MILK (SUMMER)	4 cups raw coconut water (instead of plain water) 1 cup almonds, soaked and peeled 1 vanilla bean, scraped (or 1 teaspoon vanilla extract) Pinch of salt
PISTACHIO ROSE MILK (SUMMER/FALL)	½ cup raw shelled pistachios (in addition to almonds) 1 tablespoon raw honey 1 teaspoon culinary rose water
HORCHATA (FALL/WINTER)	3–4 Medjool dates, pitted 1 tablespoon vanilla extract 1 teaspoon ground cinnamon Pinch of salt
CHOCOLATE MILK (FALL/WINTER)	¼ cup raw cacao or carob powder 3–4 tablespoons maple syrup Pinch of salt

Basic Kitchari

This simple one-pot meal is often deemed Ayurveda's "chicken soup" for its nourishing medicinal qualities. This dish is prized not only for digestive healing and cleansing protocols but also as a nourishing complete meal to be enjoyed anytime. Made from mung beans, rice, and spices, it can be a simple meal used for fasting or it can be dressed up with extra veggies and chutneys for an exciting feast. Kitchari is wonderful for all three doshas and adaptable through the seasons, so get familiar with this staple sattvic recipe and explore the many ways you can weave it into your regular repertoire.

PREP: 5 minutes | COOK: 30 minutes | YIELD: 2–4 servings

1–2 tablespoons ghee

2-inch piece fresh ginger, minced or grated

2 teaspoons ground turmeric

1 teaspoon black mustard seeds

1 teaspoon ground cumin

1 teaspoon ground coriander

1 teaspoon ground fenugreek

½ cup split mung beans

½ cup dried basmati rice

5–6 cups water

½ teaspoon salt

Lemon or lime juice, for garnish

Cilantro, for garnish

Optional: Chutney

Optional: sweet potato, pumpkin, winter or summer squash, carrots, zucchini, asparagus, or a variety of seasonal vegetables

In a medium pot, heat the ghee on low heat and add in the spices. Toast them lightly until fragrant, stirring frequently to avoid burning. Add the mung beans, rice, water, and salt. Bring to a boil. Reduce heat, cover, and allow to simmer for 25–30 minutes. For a soupier variation, continue adding water until desired consistency is reached. For a thicker stew-like variation, cook until water is mostly absorbed. Play around with adding sweet potato, pumpkin, winter or summer squash, carrots, zucchini, asparagus, or a variety of seasonal vegetables to cook into the mix. If using dense vegetables, such as root vegetables, add about halfway through cooking the kitchari and give them time to cook down. For lighter vegetables and leafy greens, steam on top in the last 5–10 minutes of cooking to keep them fresh and vibrant. Serve with a squeeze of lemon or lime juice, a heaping handful of cilantro, and a spoonful of chutney. Explore different toppings in the seasonal recipe sections of the book.

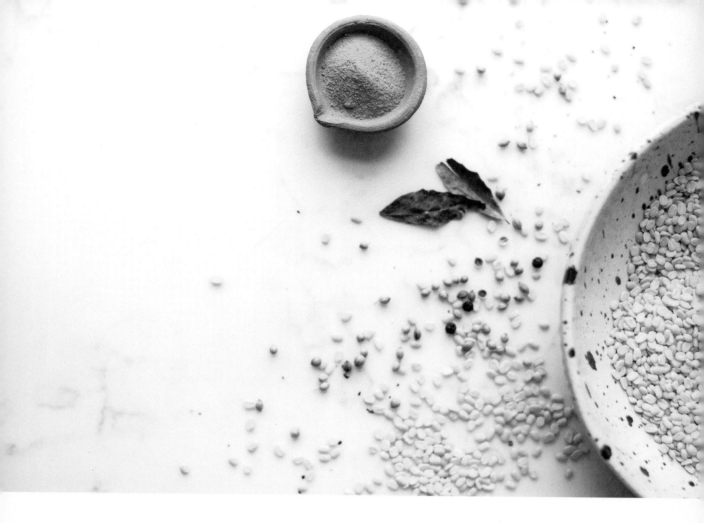

SEASONAL VARIATIONS

SPRING	8–10 asparagus stalks, trimmed and sliced into ¼-inch-thick rounds
	1 cup fresh bitter greens (arugula, dandelion greens)
	2 tablespoons lemon juice
	2 cardamom pods, crushed in mortar and pestle
SUMMER	½ medium zucchini, trimmed, quartered, and sliced into ¼-inch-thick wedges
	6 okra, trimmed and cut into ½-inch-thick slices
	1 cup spinach
	1 tablespoon lime juice
	1 teaspoon fennel seeds
FALL	1 cup cubed pumpkin, butternut squash, or sweet potato
	3–4 whole cloves
	¼ teaspoon cinnamon
WINTER	2–3 carrots, peeled and cut into ¼-inch-thick rounds
	1 cup chopped collard greens or kale
	⅛ teaspoon asafetida

Dosa

Dosas are South Indian–style crepes made from fermented lentils and rice. Don't be intimidated by the fermentation process; once you get familiar with how the process works, it becomes easy to keep a batch in rotation in your kitchen. And in a pinch, you can skip the fermentation process for a quick crepe. Dosas are versatile and can be made sweet or savory by serving with chutneys, stuffing them with vegetables, pairing along-side a curry or stew, or even pressing the batter into waffles.

PREP: 24–36 hours, soaking and fermenting | COOK: 10–30 minutes, depending on amount cooked | YIELD: About 6 cups of batter or 16 medium dosas

2 cups white basmati rice

1 cup hulled urad dal (skinless black lentils)

1 tablespoon fenugreek seeds

12 cups filtered water, divided

1 teaspoon salt

1–2 tablespoons ghee or untoasted sesame oil

Note: A heads-up—it usually takes 1–2 duds to season the pan before you start getting well-cooked dosas. Be patient and keep practicing.

In a large bowl, combine the rice, dal, and fenugreek seeds. Cover with 8 cups filtered water and soak overnight. Drain and rinse well through a fine-mesh strainer. Transfer the mixture to a high-speed blender and add 4 cups water to the total mixture. Blend until smooth. You may have to work in batches (2–3) to fit in the blender.

Pour the blended mixture into your largest bowl and stir the salt into the batter. The batter will expand during fermentation, so you want to use a bowl large enough so that it won't overflow. Cover with a cloth and place in a warm, dry area out of direct sunlight to ferment for 7–14 hours. In cool climates, the batter will take longer to ferment. If this is the case, keep it fermenting until it has a tangy, sour smell—up to 24 hours. To stop the fermentation process, give it a stir, cover with a lid, and store in the fridge for up to 3 days. Remove from the fridge and warm to room temp; be sure it is well stirred before cooking.

When ready to cook, heat a well-seasoned skillet on high heat just below smoking. Once hot, reduce heat to medium and add a little bit of ghee or untoasted sesame oil to season the pan. Ladle about ⅓ cup of the batter into the center of the pan and use the bottom of the ladle to spiral the batter from the center to evenly spread out like a thin crepe, no more than ⅛-inch thick. Cook until the batter begins to bubble and the edges curl up; the bottom will be golden but not burned. Flip and cook the other side. Remove from heat and keep warm to serve. Lightly oil the pan between dosas.

Chapati

Chapati is a simple flatbread, similar to a tortilla, made with whole wheat flour and cooked atop a hot skillet or an open flame. It's a traditional staple in a yogi's diet, often paired alongside a dal or vegetable dish with chutneys. You'll see this recipe make a few appearances as a pizza crust, a tortilla for summer tacos, and even stuffed with herbs and veggies.

PREP: 20 minutes | COOK: 5–10 minutes, depending on amount cooked | YIELD: 8 small chapatis or 4 large chapatis

2 cups whole wheat flour pastry flour, plus extra flour for dusting

1 teaspoon salt

1 tablespoon melted ghee or sunflower oil

½ cup water, plus 3 extra tablespoons if needed

1–2 tablespoons ghee

Optional: sesame seeds, spices, or chopped dates

In a large bowl, combine the flour and salt. Add the ghee or oil. Pour half of the water into the flour mixture. Begin mixing by hand, adding in more water 1 tablespoon at a time and working the mixture until it begins to form a dough. You want the dough to be firm but not too dry. If it is too wet or sticky, add a little more flour. Avoid overhandling the dough. Once formed, cover with a damp towel and let sit at room temperature for 20 minutes or longer. You can also cover and store in the fridge overnight.

When ready to use, remove from fridge, if stored, and allow the dough to warm to room temp before rolling. Prepare a cutting board or flat surface with a dusting of flour. Tear off small pieces of dough, rolling them with your hands into 2-inch balls. Using the heel of your hand, press each ball into a flat circle on the floured surface, then roll evenly with a rolling pin to a thick tortilla-like round. If you're adding special ingredients, such as sesame seeds, spices, or chopped dates, now is when you would sprinkle them across the top of the chapati and roll over once with the rolling pin to press into the dough. Gently lift the chapati off the surface so as not to tear.

Preheat a well-seasoned skillet on medium-high heat until just below smoking. Put a dab of ghee onto the hot skillet and place a chapati on top. Cook for 60–90 seconds on each side. You'll see pockets of air bubble up between the top and bottom layers and

continued

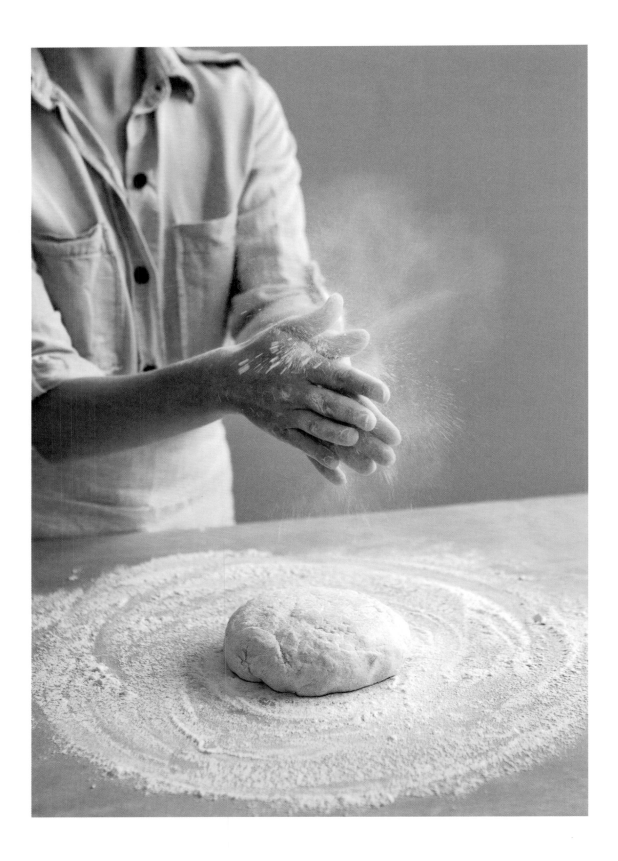

the edges will begin to crack or curl up. Flip over and cook for another minute or less, depending on how hot your pan is. A little smoking of the pan is normal when cooking these, so turn on your hood fan. Keep your eye on these because they cook fast! Store in a tortilla warmer or cover with a cloth in a pie pan to keep warm before serving.

Note: Use freshly ground flour whenever possible. It's easy to make fresh whole wheat flour by grinding whole wheat berries into a powder in a blender or grain mill. Whole wheat is nourishing for vata and pitta, while barley or rye flour can be used for kapha. For a gluten-free alternative, try 1 cup brown rice and 1 cup quinoa flour.

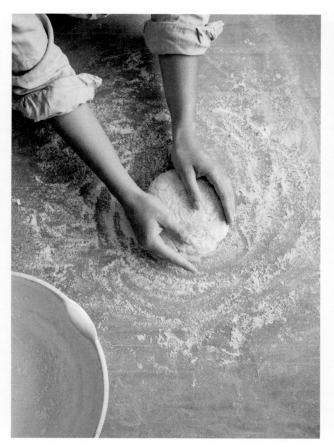
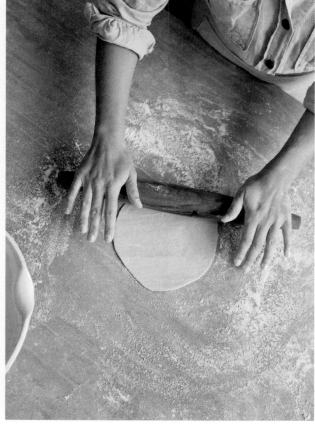

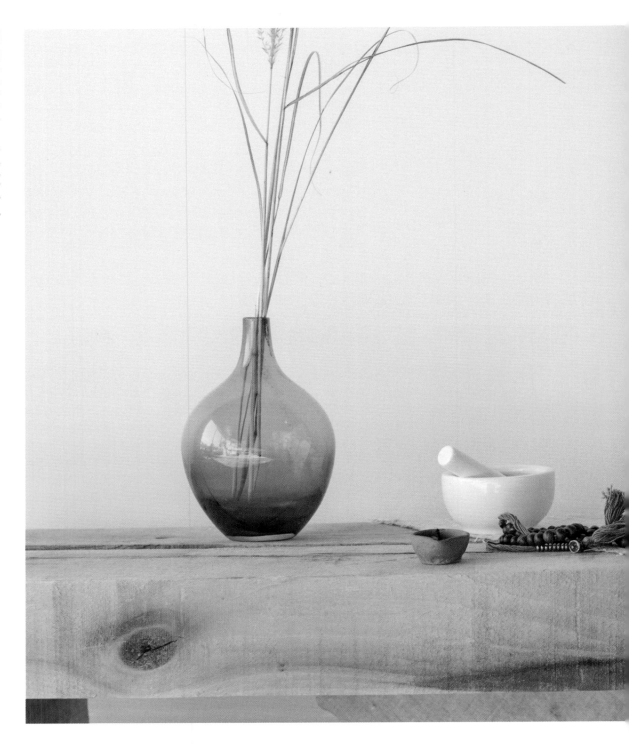

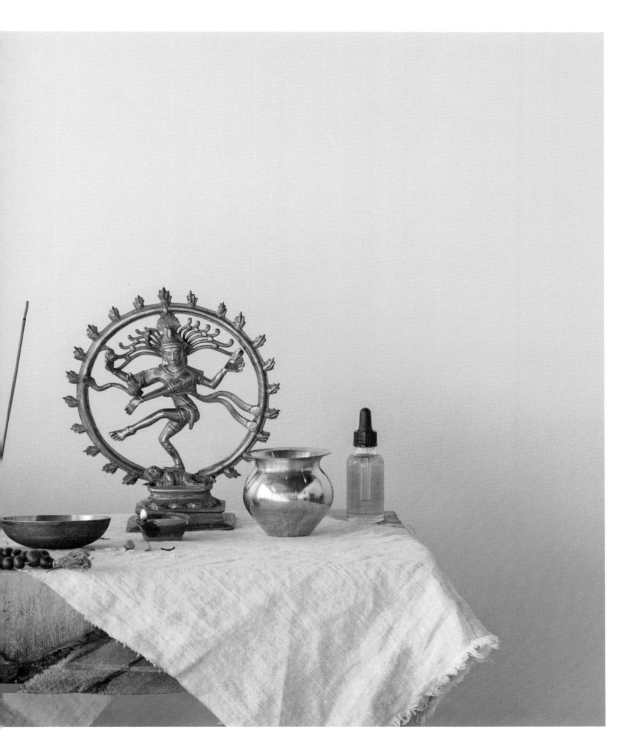

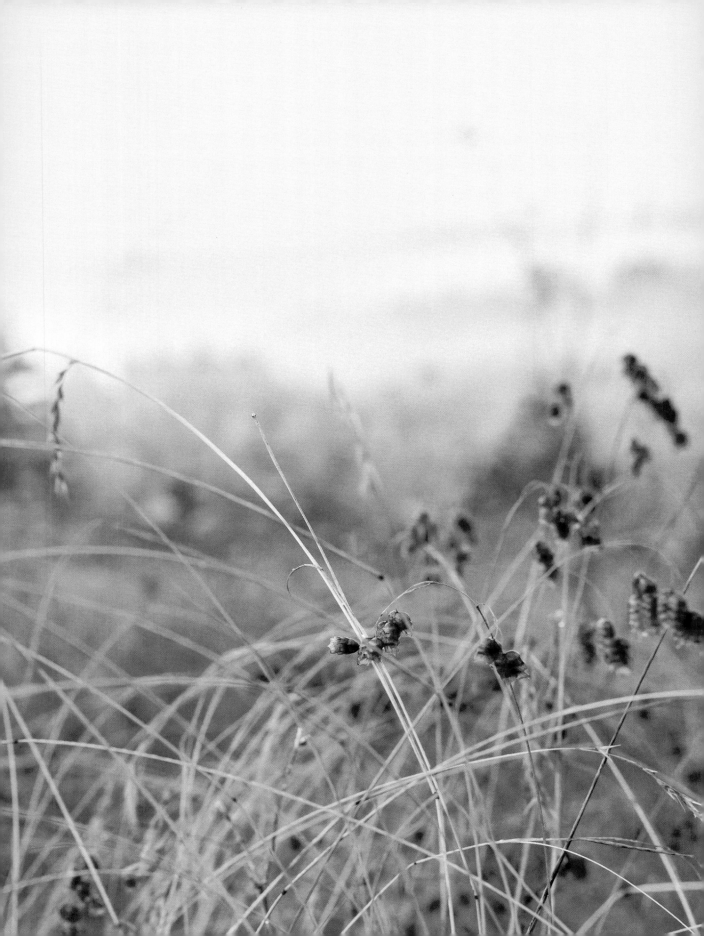

PART THREE

SPRING

Winter's snow melts, April brings cool showers. Spring has arrived.

Spring is kapha season. The heavy, slow, cool qualities and wet weather of late winter and early spring welcome a lightness into our food, breath, and movement practices to balance and brighten kapha. As we move through the seasons, we select foods and adopt a lifestyle that will reduce the increased elements of earth and water. To move out of winter's sleepy hibernation, your spring practice might include more active movement; breathing practices that bring heat and boost circulation; and lighter foods to energize the body and mind. Spring is also one of the two recommended times in the year to do a cleanse (see page 99). When you're feeling dull, heavy, or stagnant, look for ways to lighten up and breathe more vibrancy back into your routine.

Staying Balanced through Spring

EMPHASIZE

FOOD: Incorporate light, cleansing, warm, and freshly cooked foods with raw greens and sprouts, warm grains, legumes, pungent spices, bitter vegetables, and astringent herbs. Enjoy room-temp or hot beverages such as herbal teas like tulsi, dandelion, and nettle or green or black tea in small amounts.

BREATH: Focus on invigorating and energizing breath practices that break up stagnation in the chest; regular breathing that expands the lungs and rib cage and emphasizes longer exhales.

MOVEMENT: Try steady, strengthening, vigorous, and heating asana with longer-held postures. If not yoga, ask yourself in what ways can you move your body that will bring joy and a sense of vibrancy to your day.

MEDITATION: Walking meditation in nature; contemplating the vastness of the open sky; meditation should be light, lively, energizing, and expansive.

FOOD: Sugar, fried foods, overly oily or fatty foods, homogenized dairy, ice cream, meat, canned or frozen foods, cold beverages and smoothies; overeating, snacking, or grazing.

BREATH: Erratic, tight, shallow, or absent breath awareness that leads to stagnation, especially in the chest.

MOVEMENT: Inconsistent movement, oversleeping, sitting for extended periods of time, long Savasana or naps.

Tips for Tending Your Inner Fire in Spring

Spring can bring sluggish, sticky and slow digestion. If you notice these qualities, try these tips for reigniting your inner fire:

- Start the day with a large mug of hot water with lemon and ½ teaspoon raw honey to ignite digestive fire. If you wake up with low appetite, prepare a Ginger Appetizer (page 64) and chew well before your meal.

- Eat a light breakfast (like Grapefruit with Cardamom & Honey, page 109) or wait until true hunger arises for lunchtime. By noon, be sure to eat a nourishing lunch, don't skip this meal, and end the day with a light dinner. Keep your digestive fire running smooth by eating routinely and avoid mindless grazing throughout the day.

- Put down the ice water or cold smoothie. Instead, sip on warm water and try a hot cup of CCF Tea (page 65) or Ginger Fennel Tea (page 105).

- After eating, take a brisk walk outside for 5–10 minutes. More vigorous movement and sweating is helpful to counteract the sluggish tendencies of spring.

- Eat lightly one day a week, fasting on Kitchari (page 70) and herbal teas to restore digestion if you're feeling sluggish. Follow a day protocol in the Spring Equinox Cleanse (page 99) when needed.

Spring Asana: *Energizing*

Start your day with an energizing morning yoga practice. This kapha-balancing sequence focuses on dynamic movement with longer holds, chest openers, and twists to cleanse and strengthen the body. Back bending and twisting encourage opening the heart to relax and release attachments. While it's recommended to do this sequence on an empty stomach in the morning, it can also be done in the afternoon, several hours after eating. As you move through this practice, ask yourself, "Where can I create more space in my life? How can I soften my inner resistance to change?"

SPRING PRACTICE TIPS

- Prepare your practice space the night before.

- Focus on deep ujjayi breathing to warm your body while moving.

- Practice with a brisk pace to generate heat and break a sweat.

- Incorporate longer holds in postures with a focused gaze to stay engaged.

- If you're feeling resistance to movement, try the Spring Pranayama practice first (page 94) to warm up.

DOSHA NOTES

(V) Shorten holds for 1–2 breaths per posture to avoid overexerting yourself, focus on smooth and steady breathing. Enjoy a longer Savasana to support your nervous system.

(P) Move through the sequence with fluidity and repetition, holding postures for a shorter duration but repeating the overall sequence several times to satisfy the need for movement and challenge without becoming overheated. Practice with a gentle, lighthearted attitude.

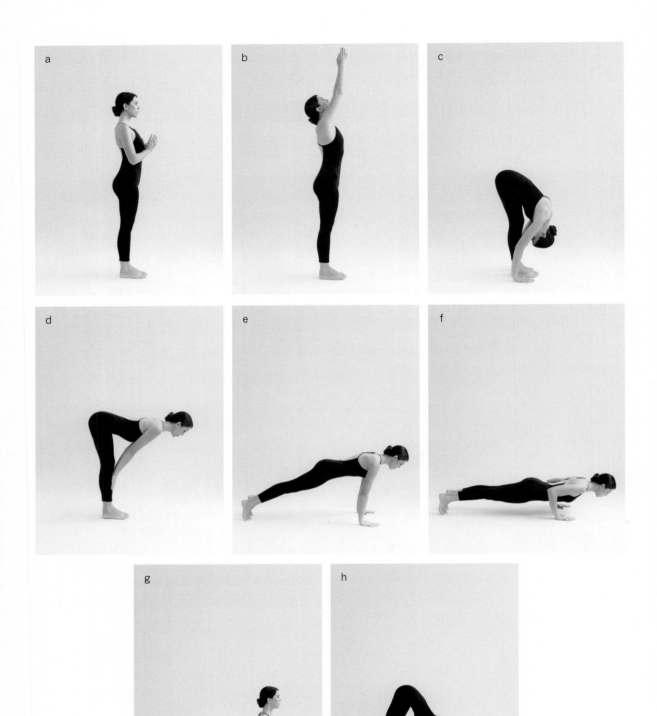

1 SURYA NAMASKAR (SUN SALUTATION SEQUENCE)

a Stand with your feet together and palms in prayer at your heart. Draw your navel inward toward your spine, lift your heart and broaden your shoulders.

b Inhale, extend your arms overhead.

c Exhale, bend slightly at your knees and lower your upper body toward your thighs to come into a standing forward fold.

d Inhale, lift your upper body and extend your spine straight, draw your hands to your shins.

e Exhale, fold forward again. Bend your knees deeply. Place your hands on the ground and step back into a plank position and hold for 5 breaths. Lengthen your spine and engage your abs.

f Exhale, bend your elbows, and hug your upper arms to your rib cage. Lower your body to the floor.

g Inhale, arch your upper back to lift your chest off the floor into a gentle back-bend. Keep your legs and feet on the pressed to the ground. Exhale, lower back to your belly.

h Inhale, press your body away from the floor in a reverse push-up, your knees can stay on the ground for support. Lift your hips upward and press your chest back toward your upper thighs, moving into a Downward-Facing Dog posture. Hold for 5 breaths.

c Exhale, step your feet forward to the front of the mat, returning to a standing forward fold.

b Inhale, raise your upper body back to standing with your arms extended overhead.

a Exhale, lower your arms and join your hands at your heart in prayer.

Repeat 3–5 times at a steady, active pace to generate heat in your body.

MODIFICATIONS

- For low back or shoulder sensitivities, always practice with your knees on the ground for a modified plank.

- For tight hamstrings, bend the knees in the standing forward folds and use blocks beneath the hands for support.

2 UTKATASANA (CHAIR POSE)

Stand with both your feet together. Draw your hands in prayer position at your heart. Inhale, stretch your arms overhead. Exhale, bend your knees and sit back like you're sitting in a chair. Lift your upper body and broaden your chest. Hold for 5 breaths. Return to standing when done.

MODIFICATIONS

Place a block between your thighs for more stability with feet hip-distance apart.

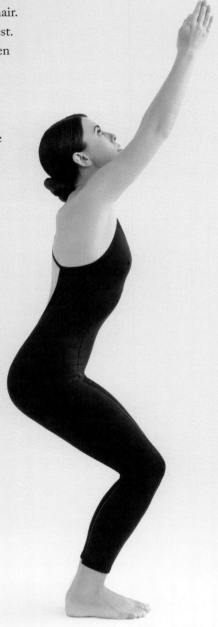

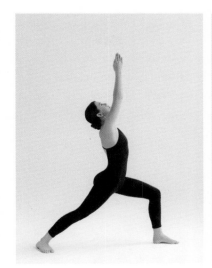 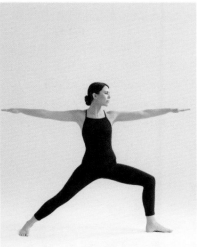

3 VIRABHADRASANA A (WARRIOR 1 POSE)

Step your left foot back about 4–5 feet at a 45-degree angle. Keep your right foot pointed forward. Bend your right knee directly over your ankle. Keep your left leg straight, pressing weight into the outer edge of the foot. Your hips will face the front of the mat. Lift your arms overhead and gaze toward your hands. Hold for 5 breaths. Return to standing when done. Repeat on the other side.

MODIFICATIONS

- For tight ankles and hips, lift your back heel off the ground into a lunge position.

4 VIRABHADRASANA B (WARRIOR 2 POSE)

Step your left foot back 4–5 feet, or as wide as your wrists when your arms are extended. Turn your foot to face the long side of the mat. Keep your right foot facing forward. Bend your right knee directly over your right ankle, and keep your left leg straight. Your hips will face the side of the mat. Extend your arms wide at shoulder height, palms facing down. Gaze over your front hand. Hold for 5 breaths. Return to standing when done. Repeat on the other side.

MODIFICATIONS

- Stand with the edge of your back foot braced against a wall for support.

5 PARSVAKONASANA (EXTENDED SIDE ANGLE POSE)

From Warrior 2 Pose, lower your right forearm onto your right thigh. If mobility allows, lower your right hand to the ground or a block placed on the outside of your right foot. Inhale, extend your left arm overhead toward the front of the mat. Rotate your shoulders open to the side of the mat. Hold for 5 breaths. Return to standing when done. Repeat on the other side.

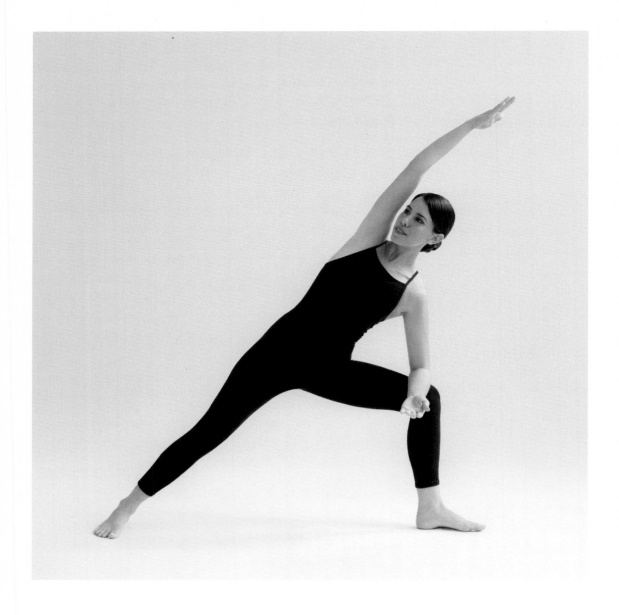

6 ARDHA CHANDRASANA (HALF MOON POSE)

From Warrior 2 Pose, lower your right forearm to your right thigh and your left hand to your left hip. Inhale, transfer your weight to your right leg and reach your right hand to the ground or a block about a foot in front of your right foot. Gaze at a side wall or the floor. Balance on your right leg and lift your left leg until it's parallel to the floor, creating a 90-degree angle in your legs. Open your body to face the side of the mat. Reach your left arm upward toward the sky. Balance and breathe. Hold for 5 breaths. Return to standing. Repeat on the other side.

MODIFICATIONS

- Use a block or chair under your supporting hand for stability or place your lifted foot against wall.

- Skip this posture if you've had a hip replacement.

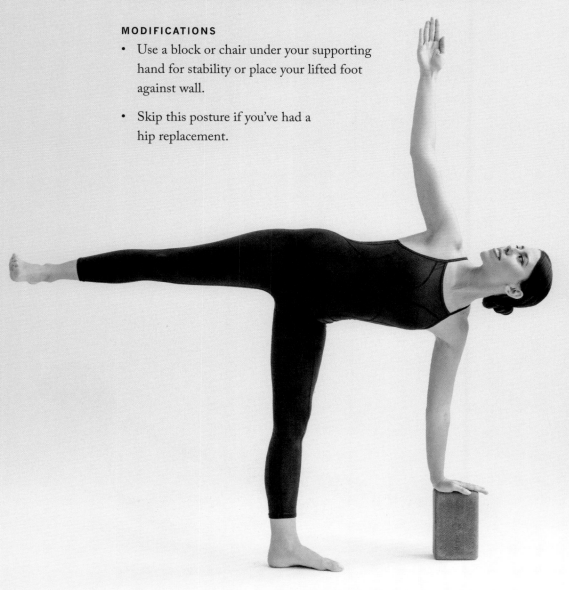

7 SALABHASANA (LOCUST POSE)

Lie onto your belly. Extend your arms by your sides and draw your legs together. Rest your forehead on the floor. Squeeze your inner thighs and press the tops of your feet to the floor to create a stable base in your lower body. Press the backs of your hands into the floor. Inhale, lift your chest and head off the floor into a gentle backbend. Hold for 5 breaths. Lower your upper body and rest with your head turned to one side. Repeat 2–3 more times. When complete, draw your hips back to your heels and release your upper body on your thighs in Child's Pose.

MODIFICATIONS

- Focus on engaging your abs and lengthen your tailbone to relieve low-back tension.

- Extend your arms forward and lift your legs for a more challenging variation.

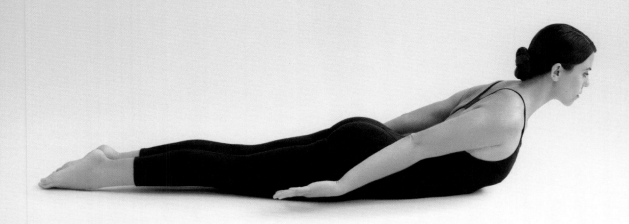

USTRASANA (CAMEL POSE)

Stand on your knees and separate your thighs hip-distance apart. Inhale, lengthen your spine and place your palms on your lower back with your fingers facing down. Exhale, draw your chin toward your chest. Inhale, strongly engage your abdominals, breathe into your sternum, and draw your shoulder blades together to arch your upper back into a backbend. Hold for 5 breaths. Return to Child's Pose to rest.

MODIFICATIONS

- Place a block between your thighs to stabilize your lower body and a blanket below the knees for sensitive knees.

- Lower your hands to your heels for a deeper backbend.

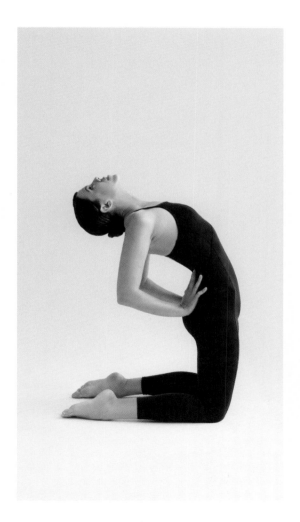
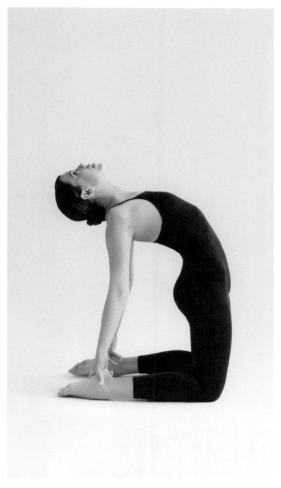

NAVASANA (BOAT POSE)

Sit upright and extend your legs in front of you. Inhale, bend your knees, place your feet on the floor, and hold behind your knees. Exhale, lean your upper body back, keeping your spine straight. Find a stable balancing point on your sit bones, lift your feet, and draw your shins parallel to the floor. Bring your big toes to touch, flex your toes, and press through the balls of your feet. Hold for 5 breaths. Lower your feet for a rest, then repeat for 3–5 times.

MODIFICATIONS

- Keep your feet on the floor for a gentle variation.

- Extend your hands and legs straight for a more challenging variation.

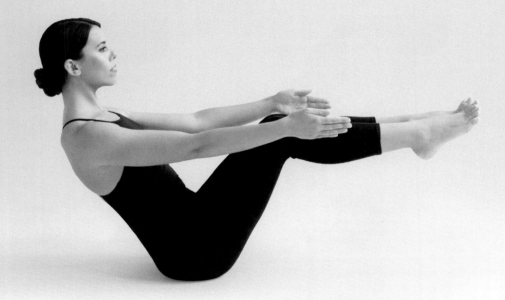

JATHARA PARIVARTANASANA (SUPINE TWISTS)

Lie flat on your back, draw your knees into your chest. Inhale, extend your arms out to your sides at shoulder height, palms facing down. Exhale, engage your pelvic floor and abs, slowly lower your legs over to the right side of your body onto the floor. Turn your head away from your legs. Hold for 5–10 breaths, with each breath easing deeper into the twist. To come out of the posture, actively engage your abs and lift your legs back to center, use your hands for support if needed. Repeat on the other side.

MODIFICATIONS

- Place a pillow or blanket between and beneath your bent knees to relieve low-back discomfort.

- Straighten one leg and twist with one knee bent.

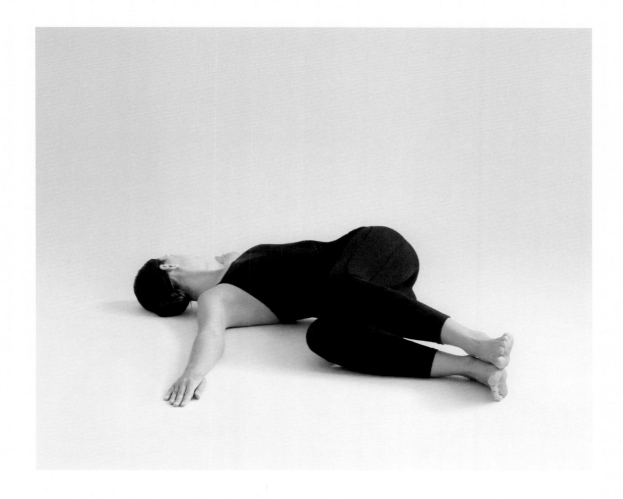

SARVANGASANA (SHOULDERSTAND)

Lie on your back, draw your knees into your chest. Press your palms into the floor and lift your hips over your shoulders. Bend your elbows and support your mid back with your hands. Draw your legs overhead, keeping your knees bent, and adjust so you're resting on the top edges of your shoulders. Lengthen through the crown of your head to draw your chin away from your chest. Straighten and lift your legs, drawing your shoulders, hips, and legs into a vertical line. Gaze at your toes. Hold for 5–10 breaths. When complete, lower your legs overhead and release your arms by your sides, using them as support to roll down onto your back. Draw your knees to your chest and rest here for a few breaths.

MODIFICATIONS

- Use 1–2 folded blankets under your upper back and shoulders to take weight off your neck.

- Skip this posture if you have high blood pressure or glaucoma, or if you are pregnant or menstruating. Instead, try lying on your back with legs against the wall for a gentle inversion.

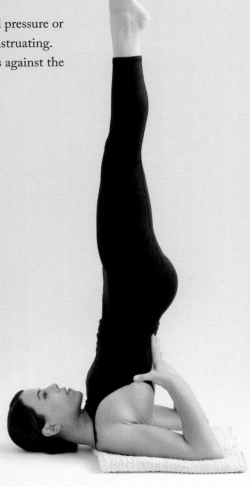

SAVASANA (CORPSE POSE)

The queen of all poses—do not skip this one! Set a gentle alarm if you're worried you may fall asleep. Lie on your back with your legs extended long and your palms resting by your side. Close your eyes, exhale deeply, and relax every inch of your body. Relax any controlled effort to breathe. Rest in stillness for 5–7 minutes to complete your practice.

MODIFICATIONS

- Place a pillow or bolster under your knees and an eye pillow/cloth over your eyes.

- Cover yourself with a blanket if you're cold.

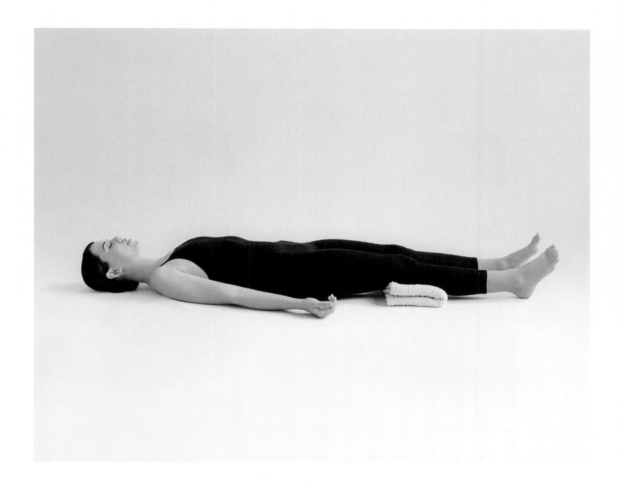

Spring Pranayama: *Kapalabhati*

Kapalabhati, sometimes called the "skull shining breath," is one of the six yogic purification practices (*shatkarmas*) used to help clear mucus out of the head and respiratory system. It's an invaluable practice for spring when the increase of water in our surrounding environment can affect and slow down our own inner waterways. There are five waters of the body governed by kapha, each influencing the stomach, heart, tongue, head, and joints, respectively. You might notice your digestion is slower this time of year, or your lungs get bogged down with fluid, making you more susceptible to head colds and feeling lethargic.

This pranayama practice is all about clearing out any stagnancy in these pathways and bringing invigorating energy back into the body and mind. It's a fairly active and heat-building breath, so you'll quickly notice a shift in how you feel after you do this practice. Because of this, it's best practiced in the morning on an empty stomach. Skip or practice softly if you're feeling overheated. If congested, try jala neti (page 50) to clear the sinuses first.

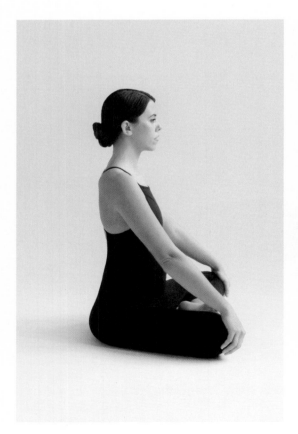 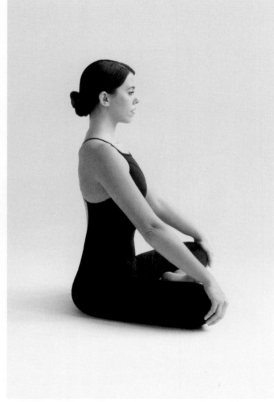

HOW TO

Many yogic breathing practices focus on the expansion and contraction of the diaphragm. In Kapalabhati breathing, you are actually focusing on contracting your belly as you exhale, followed by a passive inhalation while relaxing your abdominals. Your rib cage will move as a natural process of breathing, but let your focus rest on your navel.

1   Sit in a comfortable position that supports your spine and hips. This can be done cross-legged on the floor or upright in a chair. However you choose to sit, make sure your knees are relaxed below your hips and your spine is straight. Relax your shoulders, neck, and jaw. Soften your belly.

2   Take a deep inhale through your nose into your belly; feel your belly expand. With a sharp, quick exhale, contract your navel and press the air out of your nostrils. As you release the contraction of the belly, let your breath fill your lungs and your belly expand again. This will happen almost automatically, without forcing the inhalation. Don't try to inhale actively; simply allow the inhalations to happen between exhalations.

3   Repeat this again, slowly at first as you get a feel for this breath movement in your body. Once you're comfortable, the rhythm of your breath can be done slowly and steadily with strength as you contract your belly, or at a quick and rapid pace with more emphasis on circulating more air through your lungs.

4   As you find your pace, a full inhalation and exhalation counts as 1 breath cycle. Repeat this 20 times. End on the exhalation, then take 3 deep breaths to pause and reset. This is 1 round.

5   Repeat 3–5 rounds for a full practice.

PRACTICE NOTE

Do not do this practice if you are pregnant, menstruating, have acute asthma, epilepsy, high blood pressure, an artificial pacemaker, or a stent. If you are feeling light-headed, stop the practice and rest as needed. It is important you are sitting up straight with your ears positioned over your shoulders and your chin lifted in normal alignment, to keep your airways open.

Spring Lunar Ritual: *New Moon*

The new moon is the first phase of a lunar cycle. It's the time when the night sky is the darkest. Without the moon's light, our energy is naturally lower, and we desire more sleep and time for inward reflection. The new moon offers a moment to consciously pause, schedule less, and create space for a day or evening of inward reflection. It's an ideal time to start a cleanse, contemplate the past cycle, and observe where to direct your energy in the cycle ahead.

WOMEN'S LUNAR RITUAL

The new moon is traditionally the time of menstruation. When our bodies are synced with the rhythms of nature, we bleed and begin a new cycle with the new moon. It's also a time of deep cleansing, when we release tissues, toxins, and energy from the past cycle. During menstruation, vata increases and invites a time to slow down and rest to create nourishing stability and space for renewal. If you're used to exercising heavily, try scheduling days to rest or do restorative yoga on the first 2–3 days of your cycle. Because digestion can be weaker during menstruation, eating lightly and enjoying kitchari on these days will ease discomforts. Even if you are not menstruating on the new moon, try scheduling a rest day on the new moon itself and on the start of your own moon cycle. This very simple act can help you realign and recalibrate your inner rhythms over time.

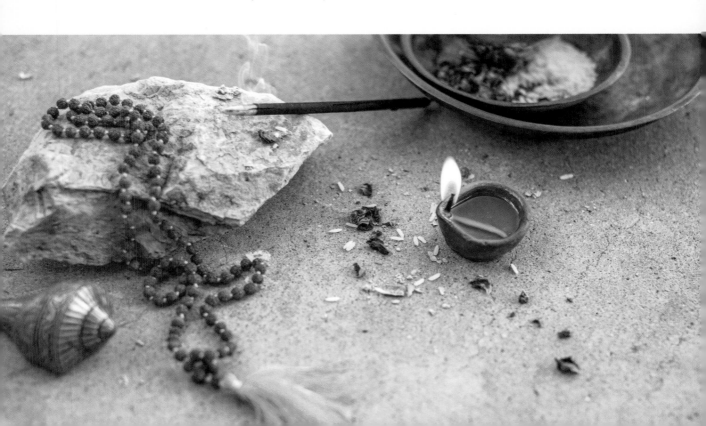

BRINGING IN THE LIGHT ON THE DARK MOON

After a long winter, the spring equinox signals a start to a new season and the new moon welcomes a new cycle. This is a powerful time for setting intentions and letting go of old patterns. The Vedic fire ceremony, Agni Hotra, is an ancient ritual for invoking our inner fire. It can transform stagnant emotions and breathe life into our intentions. This ritual can actually be done daily at sunrise and sunset. But for most of us, a monthly ritual might be more reasonable.

Traditionally, this practice is done in a copper vessel with cow dung and ghee to stoke the fire. You might be thinking this sounds a little out there. At my first ceremony, I did too! However, kits are widely available online now, and the experience is a powerful opportunity for anchoring ancient ritual in modern life. I've included more information on how to do a traditional Agni Hotra ceremony and where to order kits in the resources section (page 298). Here, I'll offer a simpler alternative that includes lighting a candle and repeating your mantras and intentions at sunrise on the day of the new moon.

WHAT YOU'LL NEED

A white unscented candle

½ teaspoon uncooked basmati rice

Fresh flowers and fruit

A meditation cushion or blanket

THE RITUAL

- Set up your ritual space in a safe area. Place the candle on a small plate or bowl and set on a low table or surface that protects the floor. Prepare a small bowl with rice to offer into the fire. Arrange the fresh flowers and fruit at your altar.

- Light the candle. Close your eyes and take a few deep breaths to center yourself.

- To begin, take the rice into your left hand. Chant the Gayatri Mantra for invoking the sun's light and the fire of creation:

  > *Om bhuh bhuvah suvah*
  > *tat savitur varenyam bhargo devasya*
  > *dhimahi dhiyo yo nah pracodayat svaha*

- Each time you repeat the word "*svaha,*" offer a few grains of rice to the flame. Once complete, offer your personal intentions or prayers into the fire. You can repeat the mantra three times, or, do a full round of 108 japa with a mala.

- Sit in silence in quiet contemplation for several minutes. Reflect on the prayers offered and the space you're creating for your intentions to come to life.

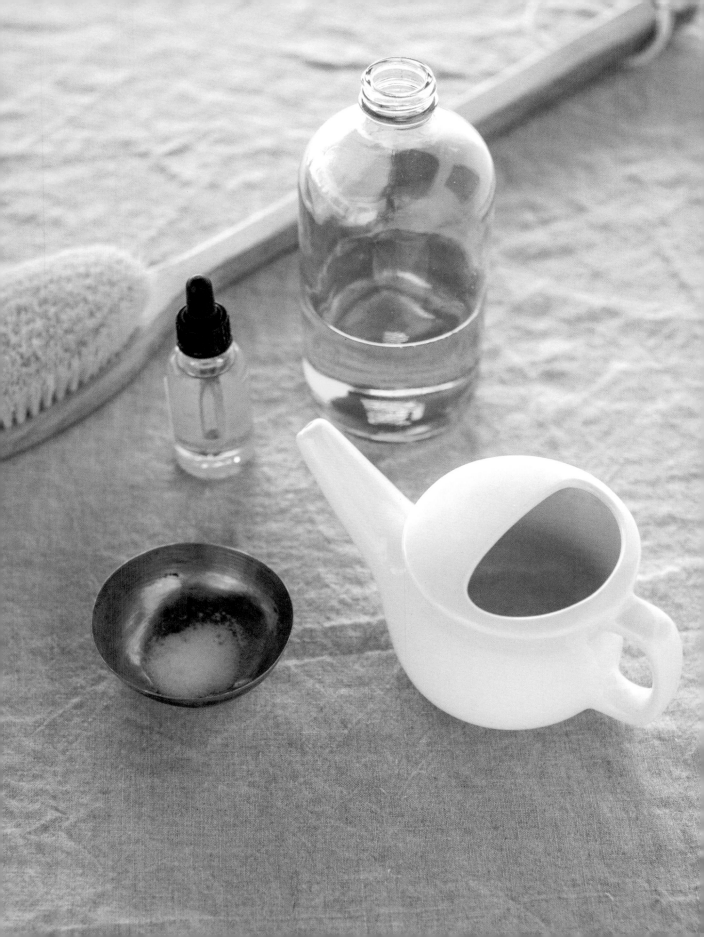

Spring Seasonal Ritual: *Equinox Cleanse*

The spring equinox pinpoints the transition from winter to spring, signaling a time to lighten up our bodies as the days start to get longer. According to Ayurveda, the junctures of the seasons are crucial times for keeping your body aligned with nature's rhythms. There are a variety of ways to fast or cleanse in accordance with the lunar and seasonal cycles. Rejuvenation practices are best performed during the waxing moon, while cleansing practices are more supported during the waning moon. So if you're choosing when to start your cleanse, plan for the time period after the full moon leading up to the new moon.

Cleansing provides a routine practice to clear out ama (unmetabolized waste or toxins) that have accumulated through the season as a result of poor diet and lifestyle choices. Ama in the mind can create mental confusion, poor memory, inability to concentrate, difficulty making decisions, lethargy, attachment, and fear. Ama in the physical body can create bloating, gas, diarrhea, constipation, indigestion, bad breath, fatigue, achy body, stiffness, and joint pain. Ama can also look like weight gain. Oftentimes excess ama will be confused with a kapha imbalance, especially in spring. It's essential to routinely clear this out in order to keep the body and mind healthy.

There are many approaches to cleansing, from a simple home cleanse to a more rigorous *panchakarma*. Panchakarma is a five-action cleansing process that includes three stages of preparation, purification, and rejuvenation to cleanse and rebuild the tissues. This protocol is best done with the guidance of a certified Ayurvedic practitioner. See the resources section (page 298) for recommended panchakarma centers. However, a simple home cleanse can be just as meaningful and impactful. Whether you're doing a longer two-week protocol or a short one-day fast, creating space to rest your senses and boost your digestion can have a profound effect on your health. This spring equinox cleanse is designed to support you, body and mind, by simplifying your diet and boosting your self-care rituals.

PREPARE

The time you take to prepare for this cleanse is just as important as the cleanse itself. First, look ahead on your calendar and block off time you can commit to your cleanse process from start to finish. The more you are able to devote to rest and reflection, the more you'll get out of the experience. I generally recommend taking a week to prepare and transition your diet. Tell your friends and family you are preparing for this experience, so they're informed and can support you along the way.

Next, spend some time cleaning out your kitchen, composting any expired food, and stocking your pantry with wholesome, organic ingredients. If caffeine, alcohol, processed foods, or sugar are a part of your regular diet, swap these out with home-cooked meals using fruits, vegetables, whole grains, and legumes as the foundation of your transitional diet. If you regularly eat animal proteins, look for good-quality sources of these products and slowly taper down the quantity you eat through the week, replacing them with more plants on your plate. Look for ways to reduce and remove inflammatory foods, thoughts, or actions that are not serving your well-being. With this in mind, craft a meal plan for your preparation week that you can confidently stick to, keeping it simple and easy to follow. Establish set mealtimes and eat 3 meals a day with no snacking in between. You'll be amazed how quickly this alone can reset the digestion!

CLEANSE

This cleanse outline can be followed for 1 day or up to 1 week. Trust your intuition on what's needed for you in this season of life. I invite you to let go of the idea of doing it all "perfectly." Instead, view this as an opportunity to breathe spaciousness into your life. If you're a seasoned cleanser, no two experiences are ever the same. Welcome in curiosity as you reconnect with yourself in a new way.

SAMPLE MENU

BREAKFAST	Spiced Amaranth Porridge with Warm Fruit Compote (page 110)
	Basic Kitchari (page 70)
LUNCH AND DINNER	Basic Kitchari (page 70)
	Grain-Free Kitchari with Fresh Beet Salad (page 126)
BETWEEN MEALS	CCF Tea (page 65)
	Ginger Fennel Tea (page 105)
	Cleansing Burdock Tea (page 108)

Your Daily Cleanse Routine

- Wake with the sun and set your intentions for the day.

- Instead of grabbing your phone, let your eyes gaze at something beautiful first—this could be fresh flowers, a yantra, a pleasing piece of art, or something in nature—stay off all technology until you finish your morning practice. Limit all media consumption throughout the day as much as possible.

- Follow your morning dinacharya routine (page 48). Promote lymphatic movement with dry skin brushing (page 51).

- Drink a large glass of warm water with 1 teaspoon fresh lemon juice and ½ teaspoon raw honey.

- Move your body. Whether with the Energizing Spring Yoga Sequence (page 81) or a brisk walk, get the energy moving in the morning and break a sweat. You may also use a steam room or sauna or take a hot bath to induce sweating.

- Prepare a pot of Kitchari (page 70) and your herbal teas for the day. Omit ghee and oils for a more cleansing meal.

- Eat at consistent times—breakfast by 8 a.m., lunch by noon, dinner by 6 p.m.

- Take time to journal, meditate, spend time in nature, and rest throughout the day.

- Wind down with a warm oil massage (page 51) and hot Epsom salt bath. Get in bed by 9 p.m. to wind down and be asleep by 10 p.m.

REJUVENATION

When you feel complete with your cleanse duration, don't forget the final stage—rejuvenation! Instead of rushing out for chocolate-covered almonds and ice cream (Yes, I've made that mistake!), use this special time to slowly reintroduce foods that are easy on your digestion. Enjoy naturally sweet foods, such as carrots, beets, fresh fruits, dates, ghee, and organic dairy, in small amounts. Spices such as saffron, cardamom, clove, and nutmeg are wonderful rejuvenating tastes for spring. Keep a journal to note how you feel. You may have noticed your senses have changed—perhaps your sense of smell is heightened or your taste buds are more sensitive. This is an invaluable time to build a strong foundation of awareness about your health and reinforce new habits.

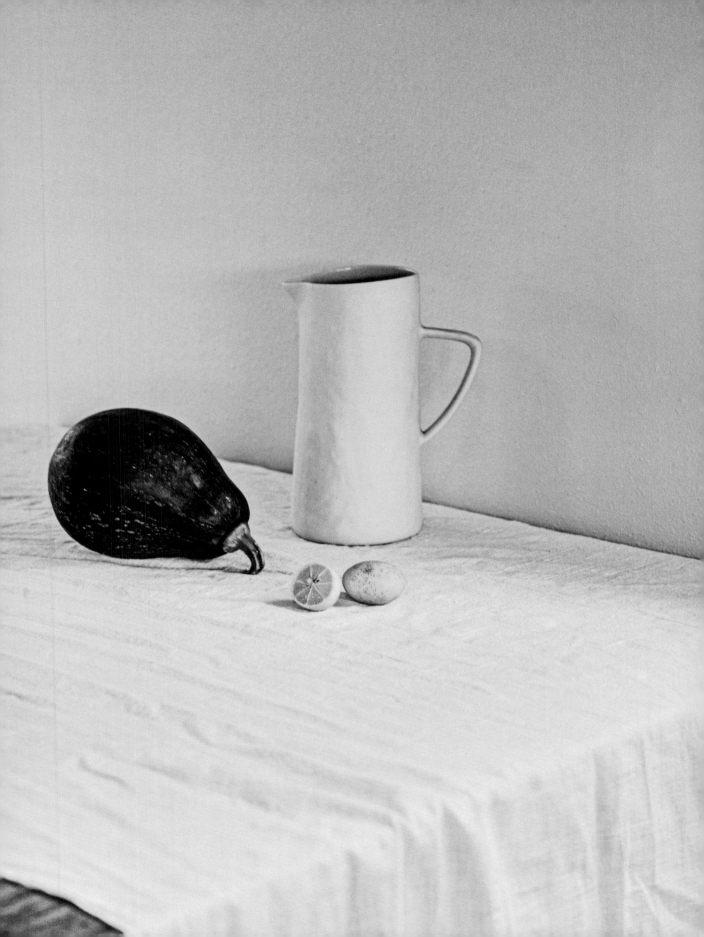

Spring Recipes

Drinks

Breakfast

Soups, Salads & Sides

Mains

Sweet

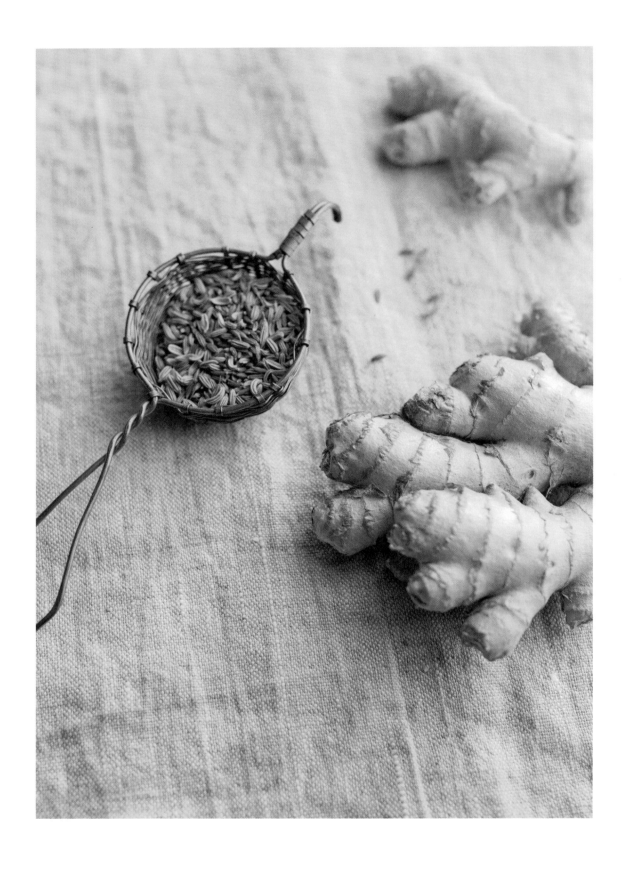

Ginger Fennel Tea

On chilly mornings when I wake up feeling a little sluggish and sleepy, I head to the kitchen and put on a pot of this tea while I start my morning routine. The windows fog up with warm condensation and the whole house smells fragrant. I like to sip a hot cup of this while I write and reflect, sometimes fasting on this until lunch, if my appetite is low. This tea is also great between meals for boosting digestion and reducing uncomfortable bloat.

PREP: 2 minutes | COOK: 10 minutes | YIELD: 4 servings

5 cups water

2 tablespoons fennel seeds

2 inches fresh ginger, roughly chopped

Optional: 1 teaspoon raw honey

In a small pot, bring water to a boil. Add the fennel and ginger. Simmer on medium heat for 5 minutes. Turn off heat, cover, and steep for another 5 minutes. Remove from heat, strain the liquid, and discard the pulp. For a little sweetness, stir in a spoonful of raw honey at the end, if desired. Sip hot, or store in a thermos to enjoy throughout the day.

A Note on Honey

Raw honey has long been prized for its beneficial nutritional and medicinal qualities, nourishing all three doshas. It's often used as a rejuvenating substance on its own, and as a yogavahi (a catalytic agent) in herbal remedies, amplifying the herbs' potency in formulations. While it has a naturally sweet taste, the aftereffect is astringent. A good-quality raw honey is loaded with beneficial enzymes. Its scraping and fat-reducing properties help reduce excess kapha. Raw is the key word here. Avoid buying any heated or processed honey. When using honey in recipes, always add in at the end after cooking. Overheating honey destroys the enzymes and makes it difficult to digest. Stir in or drizzle on top of your dish at the end for the best benefits.

Dandelion Cappuccino

Roasted dandelion root is an herbal ally in your springtime pantry. More than a common weed, this incredible herb has bitter and drying properties that reduce water retention and support your liver. It brews dark and rich, a great alternative to coffee. I like the product Dandy Blend for this recipe, it's an herbal dandelion-chicory mix that dissolves like instant coffee. Blended with almond milk and topped with cinnamon, this frothy caffeine-free cappuccino makes kicking your coffee habit easy.

PREP: 2 minutes | COOK: 1 minute | YIELD: 2 servings

1 cup water

2 tablespoons Dandy Blend

1 cup almond milk

1 teaspoon ghee or coconut oil

½ teaspoon ground cinnamon, plus extra for dusting

¼ teaspoon ground cardamom

Optional: 1 teaspoon raw honey

Bring water to a boil. Combine the Dandy Blend and piping hot water in blender. Add the remaining ingredients. Blend for 30 seconds on high until frothy. Pour into a mug, dust with cinnamon, and enjoy hot.

DOSHA NOTES

(V) Swap almond milk for organic whole or oat milk.

(P) Omit cinnamon.

What about Coffee?

Every food can be poison or medicine. Different constitutions and times of year will influence how you react to drinking a cup of coffee. For some with a vata constitution, it can create anxiety and overstimulate the nervous system. For others with a strong pitta constitution, it can create too much heat and agitation in body and mind. For those with a kapha constitution or an imbalance, the astringent and bitter tastes can actually help reduce stagnation and the diuretic qualities can balance excess water. However, coffee as a daily stimulant can lose its medicinal purpose and can actually deplete your energy over time. Check in with yourself and ask how coffee is making you feel right now. If you notice a consistent energy dip in the afternoons, try swapping your morning coffee for an herbal alternative. Sometimes all that's needed to make a graceful change is satisfying the desire for something cozy and warm in the morning.

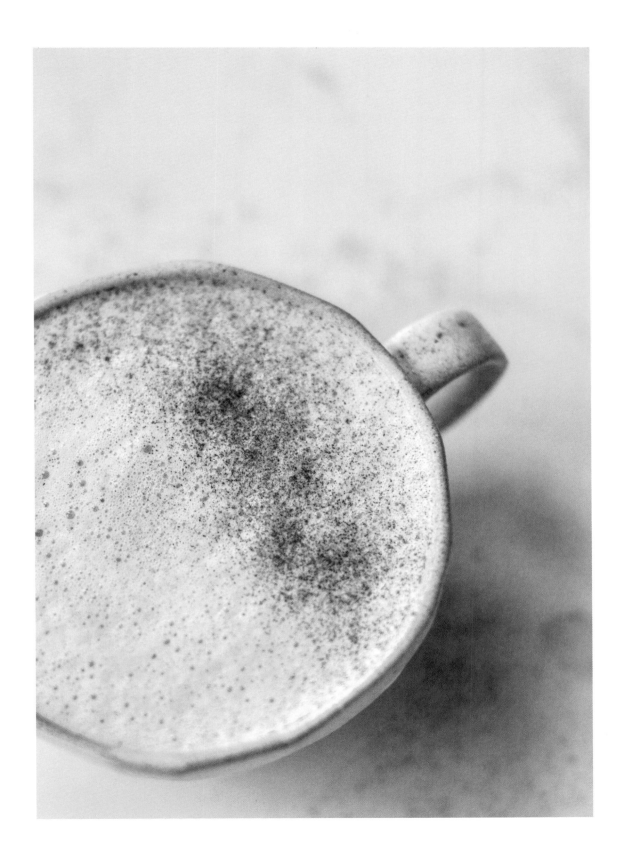

Cleansing Burdock Tea

Spring's dampness needs warming and drying properties to balance kapha. This tea combines astringent burdock with heating ginger and the sour taste of lemon to cleanse the blood and reduce water retention. Burdock has been used medicinally across cultures as a depurative, or detoxifying herb, to help remove stagnation from the lymph, flush the kidneys and liver, and improve circulation. Fresh burdock is available at many Asian markets in the produce section. I keep the dried root in bulk in my pantry to add to a tea or savory broth when needed.

PREP: 2 minutes | COOK: 10 minutes | YIELD: 4 servings

5 cups water

2 inches fresh burdock root, roughly chopped; or
2 tablespoons dried burdock root

2 inches fresh ginger, roughly chopped

2–3 tablespoons lemon juice

In a small pot, bring water to a boil. Add in the burdock and ginger. Simmer on medium heat for 5 minutes. Turn off heat, cover, and steep for another 5 minutes. Remove from heat, strain the liquid, and discard the pulp. Add lemon juice, to taste. Sip hot, or store in a thermos to enjoy throughout the day.

Alkalizing Green Juice

I hesitated incorporating juices into this book at first because I wanted to keep the kitchen equipment simple. But after a recent spring when I had felt heavy and sluggish, I remembered just how helpful having a good green juice recipe in my arsenal of medicinal drinks can be. This recipe uses bitter greens and a touch of fresh ginger to bring a little heat to the drink. Try sipping at room temperature in the morning or as an afternoon snack between meals.

PREP: 5 minutes | COOK: 5 minutes | YIELD: 2 servings

1 apple or pear

1 grapefruit, peel and pith removed

5 stalks celery

½ bunch romaine

¼ bunch dandelion greens

½ inch fresh ginger

Wash your produce thoroughly. Process all ingredients through a juicer. Pour into a glass and enjoy right away, or seal in an airtight glass container and store in your fridge for up to 36 hours.

DOSHA NOTES

Ⓥ Enjoy at room temperature.

Ⓟ Omit ginger.

Grapefruit with Cardamom & Honey

In spring, fasting or eating a light breakfast in the morning can do wonders for increasing agni and boosting metabolism. The sour and bitter tastes of grapefruit help stimulate bile production, supporting the gallbladder and liver. Try this raw for lighter meal or broiled for a warm breakfast option.

PREP: 5 minutes | YIELD: 1 serving

1 grapefruit

1 tablespoon raw honey

Pinch of ground cardamom

Peel the grapefruit and slice horizontally into thin circles. Place into a bowl. Drizzle honey and sprinkle cardamom over the top.

DOSHA NOTES

Ⓥ Broil the grapefruit for 7 minutes and drizzle with honey.

Ⓟ Omit honey.

Spiced Amaranth Porridge with Warm Fruit Compote

Cereal eaters delight. Here is a quick morning porridge that won't bog you down. If you've ever noticed feeling sleepy or sluggish after a big bowl of cereal and cold milk, a hot spiced porridge is the answer for an easy breakfast upgrade. Because like increases like, eating sugary and cold foods in the morning is a sure way to slow you down during kapha hours. Opt instead for warming, well-cooked, and easy-to-digest whole grains with supportive spices. If mornings are usually a time crunch, try making the compote the night before.

PREP: 10 minutes | COOK: 25 minutes | YIELD: Makes 2–4 servings

SPICED AMARANTH PORRIDGE

3 cups water

1 cup dry amaranth

½ teaspoon ground cardamom

¼ teaspoon ground ginger

¼ teaspoon ground cloves

Pinch of salt

Optional: milk or raw honey

WARM FRUIT COMPOTE

1 green pear, cored and cubed

1 apple, cored and cubed

½ cup raisins

6 dried figs, roughly chopped

1 tablespoon minced fresh ginger

1 teaspoon ground cinnamon

½ teaspoon ground cardamom

6 whole cloves

Pinch of ground cayenne pepper

Pinch of salt

¾ cup water

2 tablespoons orange juice

Bring the water to a boil in a small pot or saucepan. Add the amaranth and simmer for 15 minutes. Stir in the spices and salt, and cook another 5 minutes, or until the amaranth has reached a thick porridge consistency. Turn off the heat and cover to keep warm until ready to eat. To serve, top with a splash of almond milk (or milk of choice), a little drizzle of raw honey, and the warm compote.

For the compote: Combine the fruit, spices, salt, and water in a small saucepan. Bring to a low simmer and cook for 20–25 minutes, until the mixture is cooked down and sticky. If the mixture becomes too dry, add a splash of water as needed while cooking. Stir occasionally to prevent burning. Once done, squeeze in the orange juice. Taste and adjust seasonings as desired. Serve warm on top of porridge. This compote stores well in the fridge for up to 5 days.

DOSHA NOTES

Ⓥ Add 1 teaspoon ghee while cooking the porridge.

Ⓟ Omit ginger.

Millet Grits & Greens

If you're a savory breakfast eater, this whole grain–take on the classic grits is a great
way to go. Millet is a gluten-free grain that has a light and drying quality, making it a
wonderful grain for kapha. The combination of millet and brown rice together creates
a rich texture, somewhere between risotto and Southern-style grits.

PREP: 10 minutes | COOK: 25 minutes | YIELD: 2 servings

MILLET GRITS

1 tablespoon ghee or olive oil

1 teaspoon cumin seeds

1 teaspoon black mustard seeds

½ cup dry millet

½ cup dry brown rice

4 cups water

½ teaspoon salt

2–3 tablespoons fresh herbs
(rosemary, oregano, dill, basil,
parsley), finely chopped

Squeeze of lemon juice

Optional: poached or fried egg,
avocado, or fresh goat cheese

QUICK GREENS

1 teaspoon ghee or olive oil

½ bunch fresh greens (spinach,
collards, kale, chard, bok choy),
roughly chopped

Squeeze of lemon juice

Pinch of salt

In a medium saucepan, heat the ghee on medium-low heat and
toast the spices until fragrant. Stir frequently to avoid burning.
Add the millet, brown rice, and salt to the pot. Stir to coat. Add the
water and turn up the heat to bring to a boil. Once boiling, reduce
to medium heat, cover, and let cook for another 15–20 minutes. As
the water begins to cook out, stir frequently every 1–2 minutes to
fluff up the texture, until the water is fully absorbed. Remove from
heat. Taste and adjust seasonings as desired. Serve hot, topped with
quick greens, finely chopped fresh herbs, and a squeeze of lemon
juice. For a heartier breakfast, try adding an egg and a sprinkle of
fresh organic goat cheese or a few slices of avocado.

For the greens: Toward the end of cooking the grits, heat ghee on
medium in a skillet. Add the greens and stir until lightly wilted
but not overcooked, this is a quick process which takes less than a
minute. Remove from heat. Add the lemon juice and sprinkle the
salt over top. Serve hot on top of each bowl of grits.

DOSHA NOTES

(V) Enjoy with roasted root veggies or extra avocado.

(P) Swap ground coriander for the black mustard seeds.

Lemon Ginger Dal

Dal, a term for both a type of lentil and a soup dish, is a staple in an Ayurvedic kitchen. Knowing how to whip up a quick dal is a lifesaver when you're hungry and feeling uninspired on what to cook. Many Indian dals are made with tomatoes, peppers, and cream, which can be heavy and difficult to digest. My Ayurvedic approach to making dal uses a mix of savory spices, and is finished with a touch of lemon or lime to bring in acidity to balance the flavors. The result is a lighter dish that is still delicious and satisfying. I often eat this with a serving of sautéed greens and basmati rice or a chapati to round out the meal.

PREP: 5 minutes | COOK: 40 minutes | YIELD: 4–6 servings

½ cup red lentils

1 cup split yellow mung dal

1 tablespoon cumin seeds

1 teaspoon black mustard seeds

2 heaping tablespoons ghee or untoasted sesame oil

1 inch fresh ginger, minced

1 tablespoon ground turmeric

1 tablespoon ground coriander

1 teaspoon ground fenugreek

¼ teaspoon asafetida

6 cups water

½–1 teaspoon salt

1–2 tablespoons lemon juice

½ cup cilantro, chopped

In a fine-mesh strainer, rinse the red lentils and split yellow mung dal, drain, and set aside. Roughly grind the cumin and black mustard seeds in a mortar and pestle to open up the aromas, set aside.

In a large pot, heat ghee on medium-low heat. Add the fresh ginger and cook for 1 minute. Stir in the spices and heat for another minute, until fragrant. Add the red lentils and split yellow mung dal and stir until coated. Add the water and salt. Raise the heat to medium and bring to a simmer, cook for 20 minutes. Stir occasionally to prevent burning and add more water if needed. Reduce to low, cover and cook for another 15–20 minutes. Once done, add the lemon juice and cilantro. Taste and adjust seasonings as desired. Serve hot.

Note: Sometimes split yellow mung dal gets confused with split yellow peas. These are two different beans with very different cook times. Be sure you get the smaller split dal, not the larger peas!

DOSHA NOTES

Ⓥ Serve with a cooked whole grain or roasted root veggies.

Ⓟ Omit black mustard seeds.

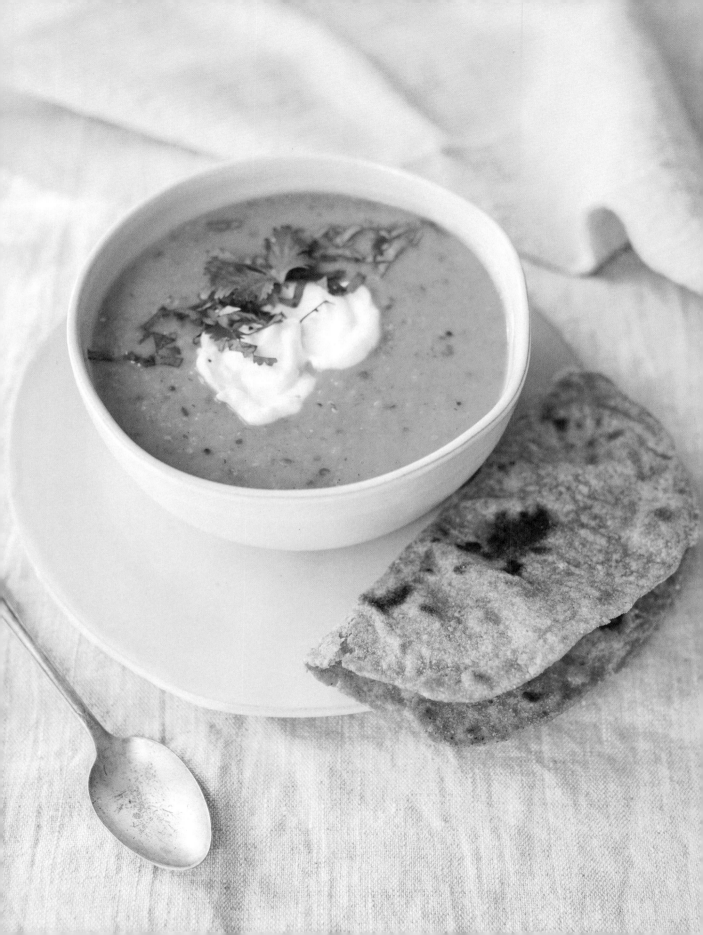

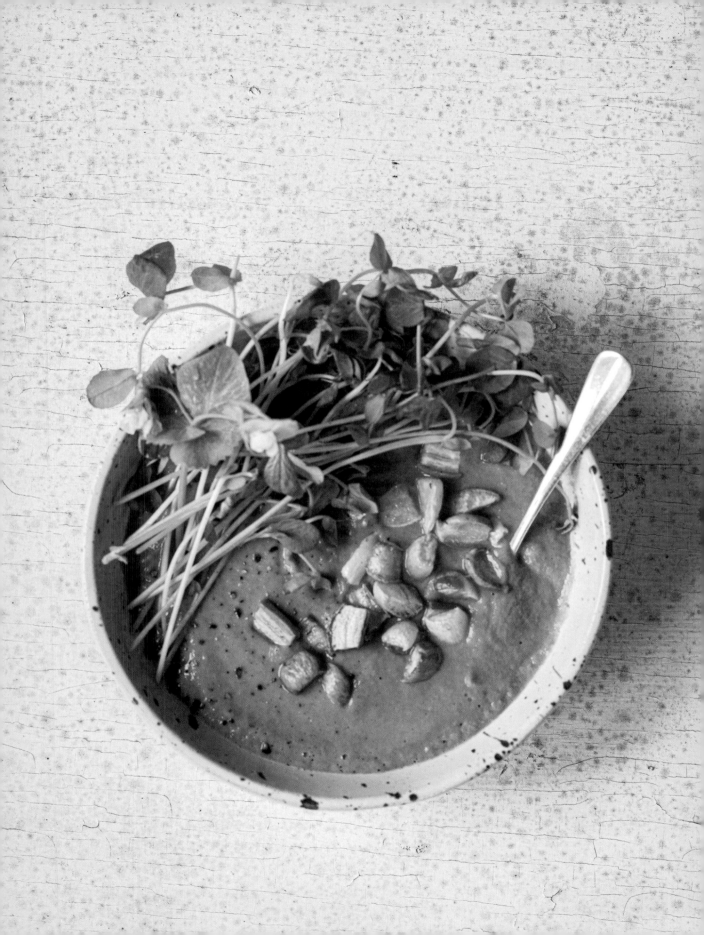

Asparagus Soup with Roasted Radishes

Radishes are an underappreciated vegetable. Cold and spicy when raw, they were always the thing I picked off a salad and set aside. I didn't really understand their value until I started cooking them—tasting them caramelized and tender, exploding with flavor after slow-roasting in the oven. They become slightly sweet and easier to digest when cooked. They're a great side dish or topping for soup. Here they add great texture and flavor alongside this light and cleansing green soup. While the radishes roast, prepare the soup.

PREP: 10 minutes | COOK: 30 minutes | YIELD: 4 servings

ROASTED RADISHES

6–8 radishes (red or French breakfast), trimmed and quartered

2 tablespoons olive oil

Salt

ASPARAGUS SOUP

2 tablespoons ghee or olive oil

1 bunch asparagus, trimmed and chopped

½ teaspoon ground coriander

⅛ teaspoon asafetida

2 cups loosely packed greens (watercress, spinach, green chard)

2–3 cups hot water

1 avocado, pitted

½ cup loosely packed flat-leaf parsley

¾ teaspoon salt

Microgreens or pea shoots, for garnish

For the radishes: Preheat the oven to 400°F. Place radishes in a baking pan. Toss in olive oil and sprinkle with salt. Roast for 20–25 minutes while making the soup, or until tender and the edges lightly browned and crispy. Remove from oven and serve hot on top of the soup.

For the soup: In a medium pot, heat the ghee on medium heat. Add the asparagus, coriander, and asafetida, and cook for 5 minutes, until tender. Reduce to low heat, add the greens, and cook another 2–3 minutes. Transfer to a high-speed blender, add the remaining ingredients, and puree until creamy, adding more water if the consistency is too thick. Taste and adjust seasonings as needed. To serve, divide between bowls and garnish with roasted radishes and a handful of microgreens or pea shoots. For a heartier meal, pour soup over a scoop of cooked quinoa or millet.

DOSHA NOTES

Ⓥ Pair with a cooked whole grain.

Ⓟ Omit asafetida.

Black Lentil, Beet & Rhubarb Salad

Where I grew up in southeast Alaska, rhubarb would sprout like weeds in our backyard in the late spring and summer months. Rhubarb is a perennial vegetable with thick, celery-like stalks that are pinkish-red in color with broad green leaves sprouting from the top. Only the root is edible when well cooked; roasting turns it into a softly sweet and sour treat. Pies and tarts are usually where you see rhubarb, but I like it for an unexpected pop of color and flavor in this springtime salad. Its sour taste pairs nicely with the astringency of the black lentils and bitterness of the fresh greens and herbs.

PREP: 10 minutes | COOK: 30 minutes | YIELD: 4 servings

SALAD

1 cup dried Beluga black lentils

4 small red beets, trimmed and quartered

2 tablespoons olive oil, divided

¼ teaspoon salt

4–5 stalks of rhubarb

2 cups arugula

¼ cup roughly chopped basil or parsley

1 cup microgreens

Soak the lentils overnight in a bowl. Rinse and drain the next day. Preheat the oven to 375°F. Toss the beets in 1 tablespoon of olive oil and a sprinkle of salt, and spread them across a baking pan. Pour a ½ cup water onto the tray and cover with foil or parchment paper to steam while cooking. Roast in the oven for 20 minutes, then remove the covering and continue to cook another 10 minutes until tender and slightly crispy outside.

Trim the ends of the rhubarb. Cut in half horizontally so the sticks are about 4-inches long, then slice vertically into ½-inch-thick sticks. Line a baking sheet with parchment and arrange the rhubarb on top. Coat in 1 tablespoon olive oil and sprinkle with a pinch of salt. Roast in the oven for 10–12 minutes, until tender but not mushy.

While the beets and rhubarb roast, drain the water from the lentils and rinse well before cooking. Fill a small pot half way with water, bring to a boil. Add the lentils and a pinch of salt, and cook for 8–12 minutes, checking the texture of the lentils to make sure they're still firm and not overcooked—you want them on the al dente side versus mushy. Soaking your lentils overnight will also decrease the actual boil time, so be mindful of how fast they're cooking. Once done, remove from heat, pour off the excess hot water, then rinse in cold water. Drain in a colander for 1–2 minutes. Transfer to a large mixing bowl. Set aside and allow to cool until ready to assemble.

VINAIGRETTE

¼ cup olive oil

3 tablespoons lemon juice

1 tablespoon lemon zest

1 small clove garlic, grated or minced

1 teaspoon raw honey

½ teaspoon ground coriander

¼ teaspoon sea salt

Pinch of ground clove

Fresh cracked black pepper

For the vinaigrette: Combine all ingredients in a jar and shake until well combined. Set aside until ready to use. This will keep in the refrigerator for 1–2 days if made in advance.

To assemble: combine the cooked lentils, cubed beets, rhubarb, arugula, and herbs in the mixing bowl. Toss with vinaigrette until lightly coated. Serve with a small handful of fresh microgreens on top.

DOSHA NOTES
Ⓥ Enjoy the salad warm.
Ⓟ Omit garlic.

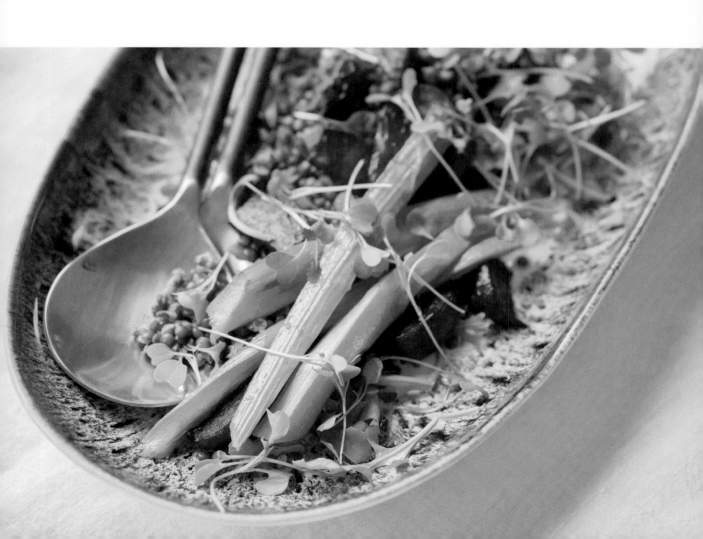

Simple Mung Sprout Salad

There's a moment around late winter and early spring when all the roasted root vegetables and stews have lost their appeal and my body yearns for something fresh and alive. Sprouts are the answer. A plant's most nutrient-rich stage of life is from germination to the first seven days of its sprouting. When we eat these little guys, they pack a fresh punch of prana and protein to our bodies. Eating live foods such as sprouts brings a welcomed lightness to the body after a long winter. And they're oh-so-easy to make once you get in the rhythm at home.

PREP: 2–4 days for sprouting | COOK: 2 minutes | YIELD: 4 servings

1 cup sprouted mung bean

2–3 tablespoons olive oil

2–3 tablespoons lemon juice

1 teaspoon sea salt

Pinch of cayenne pepper

Rinse the sprouted mung beans and pat dry with a towel. In a medium bowl, combine the fresh sprouts, olive oil, lemon juice, salt, and cayenne. Toss until well coated. Taste and adjust flavors as desired. While this can be eaten alone, this mung bean sprout salad is best enjoyed in small amounts alongside a balanced bowl.

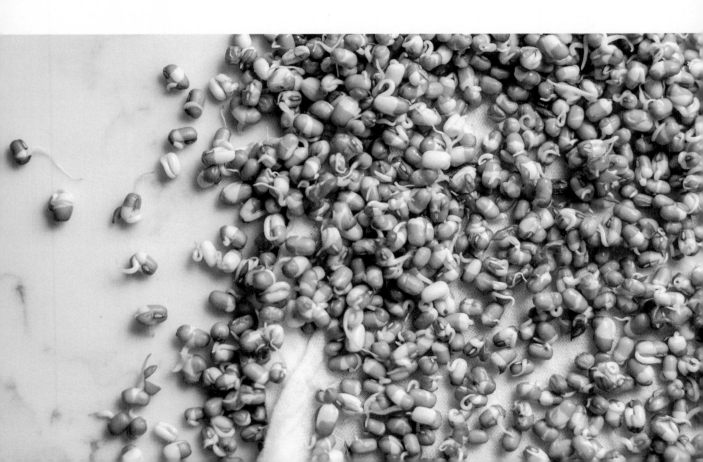

How to Sprout Anything

Have you ever noticed feeling bloated or heavy after eating canned beans or dry nuts? This is because all raw legumes, grains, nuts, and seeds contain phytic acid, a compound our bodies lack the enzyme to digest on our own. When we consume phytic acid, our bodies can't absorb essential minerals such as calcium, magnesium, zinc, and iron. Simply said: we want to soak, sprout, and cook these foods to optimize their available nutrition. Each bean, grain, nut, and seed has a different length of time needed for soaking and sprouting. There are two methods for sprouting: the tray method and the jar method. To get started, select what you would like to sprout—alfalfa, broccoli, chickpeas, fenugreek, lentils, mung beans, quinoa, radishes and sunflower seeds, to name a few ideas. Note, most nuts will not grow tails, but soaking them still increases their digestibility.

For tray sprouting: First place the beans in a large bowl, cover with filtered warm water, and let soak overnight. If the beans absorb all the water, add more to cover. The next day, drain and discard the soaking liquid. Rinse the beans once more with cold water and drain. Line a baking sheet with paper towel. Spread the beans evenly on the prepared pan, cover with a towel, and set the pan on a counter out of direct sunlight for another day to allow the beans to begin to sprout. If the beans are not sprouting after 24 hours, rinse once more under cold water. Line the baking sheet with fresh paper towel and spread the beans out again. This process may take between 36 and 48 hours total, depending on how warm and humid your kitchen is. When ready, the beans will be soft and will have grown little white tails. When ready, give them a good rinse, then spread them to dry across a towel, patting dry any extra water. Store dry sprouts in a jar in the fridge for up to 10 days.

For jar sprouting: You'll need a large glass mason jar, a metal lid, and a piece of cheesecloth. Place the seeds in the bottom of the jar, fill the jar with filtered water, cover with the cheesecloth and lid. Soak overnight. The next day, drain the water through the cloth and rinse with fresh water. Drain and allow to sit for 24 hours. Repeat the rinse and drain process again over the next 2–3 days, until tails begin to grow from the seeds and the sprouts begin to fill the jar. Store dry sprouts in a jar in the fridge for up to 10 days.

GRAIN	SOAK TIME	SPROUT TIME
Alfalfa	5 hours	3–5 days
Broccoli	8 hours	2–4 days
Chickpea	12 hours	2–3 days
Fenugreek	6 hours	2–4 days
Mung	12 hours	2–3 days
Quinoa	6 hours	1–2 days
Sunflower	8 hours	1–2 days

Spring Pea & Mung Bean Fritters with Herbed Yogurt Sauce

Ayurvedic eating doesn't have to be just dal and rice. Fritters are a fun and versatile way to work in seasonal vegetables and spices into a dish without the texture of a porridge. I'm a big fan of fritters, and you'll find a few variations peppered throughout the book.

PREP: 15 minutes | COOK: 20 minutes | YIELD: 4 servings

SPRING PEA & MUNG FRITTERS

½ cup mung flour or chickpea flour, plus 2 tablespoons

3 cups fresh or frozen spring peas, shelled

2 tablespoons tahini

2 tablespoons olive oil

4 spring onions, trimmed and finely chopped

2 tablespoons lemon juice

2 tablespoons lemon zest

2 tablespoons cilantro, finely chopped

1 teaspoon ground coriander

1 teaspoon salt

1–2 teaspoons ghee or sunflower oil, for frying

Fresh greens, for garnish

HERBED YOGURT SAUCE

½ cup plain organic yogurt (whole milk cow, goat, or coconut)

1 tablespoon cilantro, finely chopped

1 teaspoon lemon zest

½ teaspoon ground coriander

⅛ teaspoon salt

To make the mung flour, blend 1 cup of whole green mung beans in a dry high-speed blender or home grain mill. Store the flour in an airtight jar in your pantry for up to a month until ready to use. Chickpea flour makes an easy store-bought alternative to mung flour.

For the fritters: Bring water to a boil in a medium pot and blanch the peas for 3–4 minutes. Drain the peas through a sieve and pat off the excess water. Set aside 1 cup of peas and transfer the rest to a food processor. Add the remaining ingredients. Pulse a few times until mixture breaks down into a thick paste. Pulse again to incorporate the remaining cup of peas to add texture. If the mixture is too wet, add in additional flour 1 spoonful at a time. Use an ice cream scoop to portion out the patties. With wet hands, shape into balls about 2 inches wide, then flatten into ¾-inch-thick disks.

In a well-seasoned skillet, heat 1 teaspoon of ghee or sunflower oil on medium heat, just below smoking. Fry the fritters for 2–3 minutes on each side, until they are golden and crispy; use a greased spatula to flip the fritters. Cook just 1–2 at a time to avoid overcrowding in the pan. Place on a plate lined with a paper towel to absorb the oil. Serve hot with fresh greens and spoonful of the yogurt sauce.

For the yogurt sauce: Combine all ingredients in a bowl. Mix until well combined. Taste and adjust flavors as desired.

DOSHA NOTES
Ⓥ Serve with cooked greens.
Ⓟ Omit the spring onions.

Cooking with Onions & Garlic

The allium family includes onions, leeks, shallots, scallions, garlic, and the like. For many, onions and garlic are a mainstay in cooking. Looking at the six tastes, alliums are predominantly pungent, meaning they are heating and stimulating in effect. A yogic diet tends to avoid all alliums, as they are considered too rajasic and said to aggravate the mind, making meditation more challenging. Similar to coffee, it's important to notice how these foods affect your body and mind and to consume mindfully. A small amount can be great in colder weather or during rainy spring. But if you're feeling overheated or agitated, better to limit their use and opt for spices that add flavor to a dish but have a more sattvic effect on the mind. Try asafetida, sometimes called hing, a fragrant resin from the fennel plant that has a similar smell and taste as garlic. It's often used with legumes to increase digestibility and reduce their gassy effects. Add a tiny pinch to a dish and explore the flavors. A warning here: a little bit goes a long way!

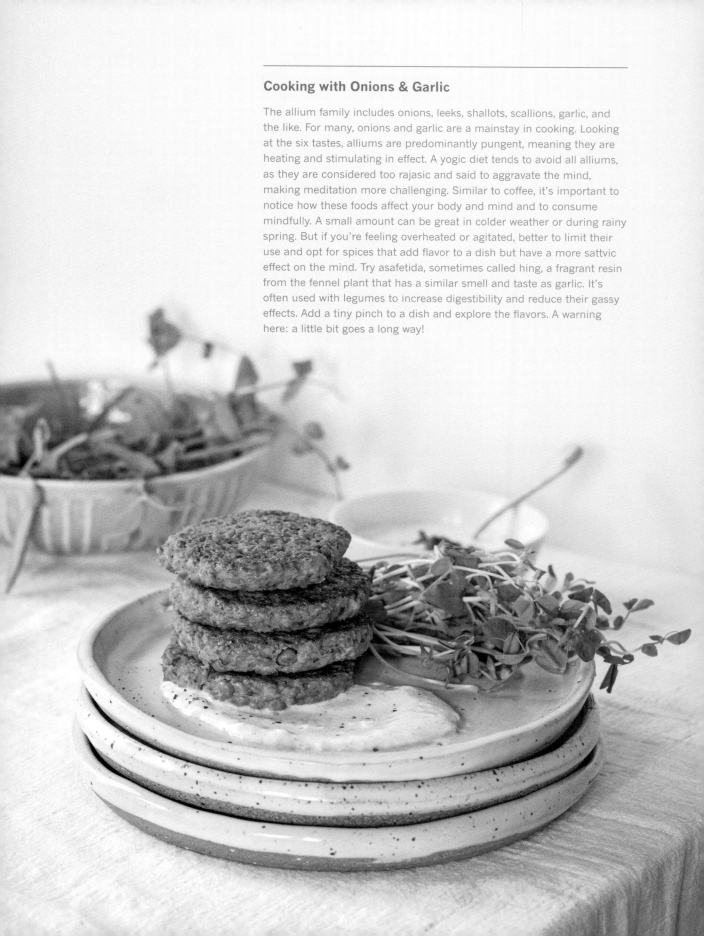

Spring Barley Risotto

It always amazes me how versatile a single ingredient can be depending on the cooking method. Take rice, for example. Every culture has its own unique preparation, from a sticky sushi rice to fluffy basmati in a biryani. But if you coat rice first in a little fat and acid, then slowly add the water over time . . . you end up with risotto, as the Italians have created. Typically made with white wine and a hearty serving of grated parmesan, this lighter spring variation uses the same cooking methods but with kapha-friendly ingredients—pearled barley, a touch of ghee, and citrus.

PREP: 2 hours | COOK: 25 minutes | YIELD: 4–6 servings

5–6 cups vegetable stock

2 tablespoons ghee or olive oil

1 shallot, chopped finely

2 cloves garlic, minced

2 cups dried pearled barley, soaked 2 hours

1 bunch asparagus, trimmed and chopped into ¼-inch rounds

2 tablespoons lemon juice

1 teaspoon salt

2 cups arugula

½ cup loosely packed parsley, finely chopped

¼ cup loosely packed mint, finely chopped

Optional: 1–2 ounces goat cheese

DOSHA NOTES
Ⓥ Increase the ghee.
Ⓟ Reduce the garlic.

In a small saucepan, bring the vegetable stock to a boil on high heat, then reduce heat to low to keep the stock warm. Starting with a hot stock is the secret to a quicker-cooking, creamier risotto. Adding in cold stock on top of the hot grain takes longer to warm up in the risotto pan and shocks the grain into holding on to its starches.

In a separate saucepan, heat the ghee on medium heat. Add the shallot and sweat in the pan for 3–5 minutes, until translucent. Add the garlic and cook for another 2–3 minutes, until golden, stirring frequently to avoid sticking or burning. Add the barley, stir until well coated, and toast in the hot pan for another 2–3 minutes. Begin to add the hot stock into the barley incrementally, pouring the broth one ½ cup at a time, stirring regularly to incorporate the liquid into the barley. Wait until the liquid has almost completely absorbed before adding another ½ cup. Be patient in this process. This gradual addition of liquid is key to getting the grain to release its starch and create that creamy texture. Ideally you want to use just enough broth to cook the barley, and no more. After about 15 minutes, the texture will start to become like a porridge, but you want the barley slightly firm—al dente, not mushy. Continue this process of adding and stirring until you reach the desired consistency; you may not use all the broth. At the end, stir the asparagus, lemon juice, and salt into the hot barley. Turn off the heat, add in the arugula and herbs. Garnish with goat cheese, if using. Serve right away while it's hot.

Green Tea Broth Bowl

Ochazuke—cha meaning "tea" and *zuke* meaning "submerged"—is a simple, warming broth bowl made from green tea poured over rice, greens, and salmon. Green tea is slightly bitter and astringent in taste and is a great ally for lightening up the dense kapha qualities in spring. Buckwheat noodles make a quick and light alternative to rice. I love this light broth bowl because it works for breakfast, lunch, or dinner. The traditional salmon or a poached egg in place of tofu makes a lovely variation, too.

PREP: 10 minutes | COOK: 15 minutes | YIELD: Makes 2 servings

TOFU

1 tablespoon toasted sesame oil

1 tablespoon tamari

2 teaspoons coconut sugar

2 teaspoons lime juice

½ teaspoon lime zest

8 ounces extra-firm organic tofu, cut into 1-inch cubes

BOK CHOY

2 heads baby bok choy, washed, trimmed, and quartered

1 tablespoon toasted sesame oil

NOODLES

2 ounces (about ½ package) dried buckwheat soba noodles

Preheat the oven to 350°F. In a small bowl, whisk together the oil, tamari, sugar, lime juice, and lime zest. Lay out the tofu cubes across a single layer of paper towel. Cover with another layer of paper towel and gently press down to absorb some of the excess water. Line a baking sheet with parchment paper, arrange tofu on the baking sheet, and pour the marinade over the tofu. Bake for 15–18 minutes to toast the tofu until slightly firm and golden on the faces. Check halfway through and shake the baking sheet to turn the cubes and prevent burning. Remove from oven and set aside.

Lightly coat the bok choy in sesame oil. Arrange on a baking sheet. Bake for 10 minutes, until tender and wilted. Remove from the oven and serve hot.

While the bok choy bakes, bring a large pot of water to a boil. Add the soba noodles and give them a stir to make sure they're fully submerged. Let the water return to a boil, then reduce the heat to a low simmer. Let the noodles cook until tender, about 6 minutes. While cooking, prepare a big bowl of cold water and a colander. When the noodles are well cooked but not mushy, drain them into the colander and then promptly dump them into the bowl of cold water. Use your hands to move the noodles around the cold water, washing off the excess starch to prevent the noodles from sticking. Drain again through the colander, letting them sit for a minute to allow excess water to drip off.

continued

BROTH

2 cups boiling water

2 tablespoons loose-leaf green tea, such as genmaicha or sencha

1 tablespoon ume plum vinegar

½ teaspoon toasted sesame oil

2 teaspoons lime juice

TOPPINGS

2 scallions, thinly sliced

¼ cup microgreens

1 teaspoon gomashio or sesame seeds

For the broth: In a French press or tea pot, pour the boiling water over the tea. Steep for 1–2 minutes. Transfer to a pot and add in the ume plum vinegar, sesame oil, and lime juice. Keep warm on the lowest heat on your stovetop. Ladle the hot broth over the bowls when ready.

To serve: use a fork to curl the soba noodles and arrange them in the bowls. Place the bok choy on top and the tofu next to it. Pour the hot tea broth over top and sprinkle with chopped scallions, microgreens, and gomashio. Serve hot.

DOSHA NOTES

(V) Try kukicha tea for a low-caffeine broth.

(P) Omit scallions.

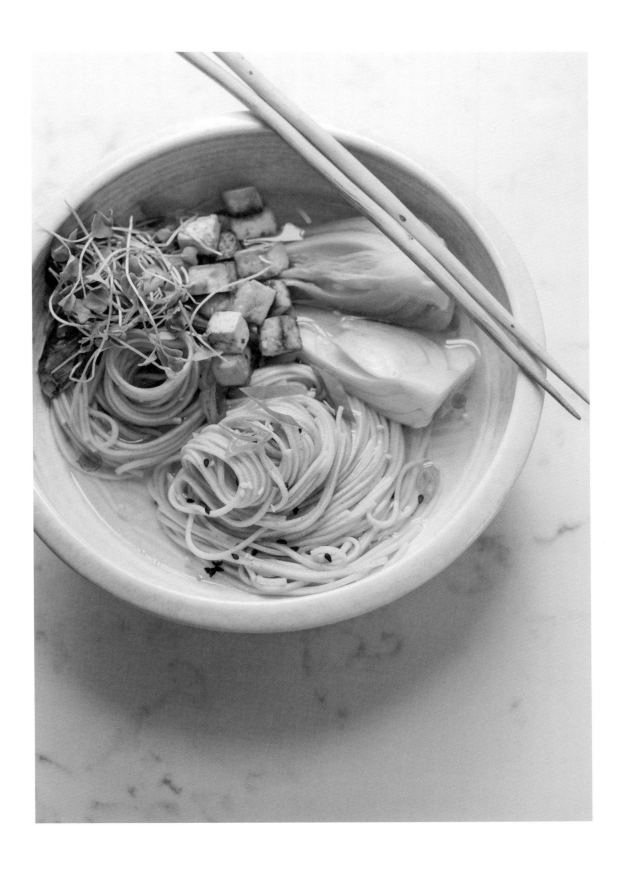

Grain-Free Kitchari with Fresh Beet Salad

When grains feel too heavy to eat, this light and flavorful grain-free kitchari is a great option for a cleansing meal. This recipe uses kapha-balancing buckwheat, which is actually a seed, not a grain. Add nutrients and flavor by using kombu, a seaweed, to lighten up on the salt. Try this topped with a fresh beet salad to help cleanse and purify the blood.

PREP: 5 minutes | COOK: 30 minutes | YIELD: 2–4 servings

KITCHARI

½ cup red lentils

½ cup split yellow mung dal

½ cup buckwheat

1 teaspoon cumin seeds

1 teaspoon black mustard seeds

4 whole cloves

1 teaspoon ground turmeric

¼ teaspoon ground cardamom

1 tablespoon ghee

2 inches fresh ginger, minced

1 3-inch piece kombu

6 cups water

¼ teaspoon salt

2 tablespoons lemon or lime juice

¼ cup cilantro, roughly chopped

Optional: fresh greens (spinach, chard, dandelion greens)

FRESH BEET SALAD

2 small red beets, scrubbed and peeled

4 tablespoons cilantro, roughly chopped

1 tablespoons fresh lemon juice

¼ teaspoon salt

In a fine-mesh strainer, rinse the red lentils, split yellow mung dal, and buckwheat. Roughly grind the cumin seeds, black mustard seeds, and cloves in a mortar and pestle. Measure out the ground turmeric and cardamom to add to the pot when ready to cook.

In a large pot, add the ghee and turn the heat to medium-low. Add the fresh ginger and stir for 1 minute, until fragrant. Next, stir in the spices and heat for another minute. Add the red lentils, split yellow mung dal, and buckwheat, and stir until coated. Add the 6 cups water, kombu, and salt. Raise the heat to medium and bring to a simmer. Cover and cook for 15 minutes at medium heat. Stir occasionally to prevent burning, add more water if needed. Reduce to low and cook for another 15–20 minutes. Once done, add the lemon juice and cilantro. You can also stir in fresh greens here, such as spinach, chard, or dandelion greens. Taste and adjust seasonings as desired. Serve hot with the fresh beet salad on top.

For the beet salad: In a small mixing bowl, use a grater to shred the beets. Add the chopped cilantro, lemon juice, and salt. Taste and adjust flavorings as desired. Serve fresh on top of the kitchari.

DOSHA NOTES

(V) Steam the beets whole before grating.

(P) Omit black mustard seeds.

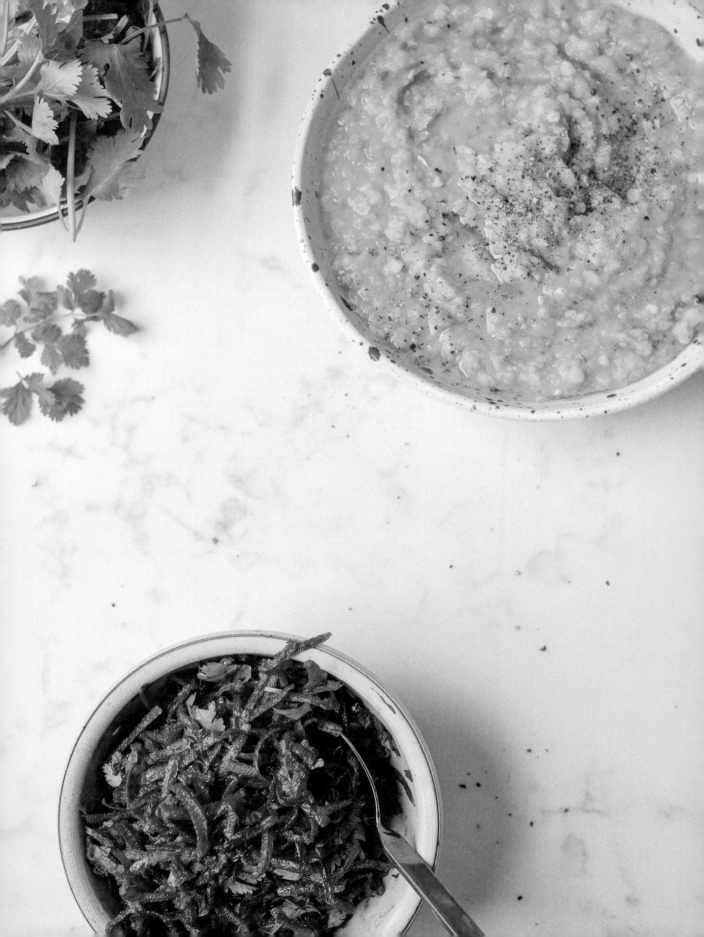

Dosa Waffles with Savory Chutney

I've been making dosas for years, but always in the traditional pancake style I learned in South India. I was delighted when I discovered dosa waffles are a real thing! After I ferment the batter, I keep it jarred and stored in the fridge for when I want to make a quick dosa to serve alongside a lunch or dinner. But some days I get fancy and pull out the waffle maker. You can even add shredded and sautéed vegetables to your batter for a denser waffle. I make the chutney in advance, to have on hand for a variety of meals. The chutney also pairs nicely with kitchari and other balanced bowl combinations.

PREP: 2 days for dosa batter | COOK: 20 minutes | YIELD: 4 servings

WAFFLES

2 cups Dosa batter (page 72)

1 tablespoon ghee or sunflower oil

Optional: sautéed spinach and poached egg

SAVORY CHUTNEY

½ cup shredded unsweetened coconut

1 bunch cilantro, including stems

½ inch fresh ginger, roughly chopped

1–2 tablespoons lime juice

½ teaspoon ground coriander

½ teaspoon black mustard seeds

½ teaspoon salt

½ cup water

Preheat the waffle maker and grease lightly with ghee or sunflower oil. Ladle out ¼ cup batter into each waffle mold and cook the waffles according to the instructions of your waffle maker. It should take between 1½ to 2 minutes depending on your waffle maker. Once done, remove from the waffle maker and serve with the chutney. For a heartier meal, add sautéed spinach and a poached egg.

For the chutney: Combine all ingredients in a high-speed blender. Blend until creamy. Taste and adjust seasonings as desired. Store in an airtight jar in the fridge for up to 5 days.

Polenta Tea Cake

Cornmeal has drying and heating properties, making this a kapha-friendly baking ingredient, especially when paired with fennel. If you have a sweet craving in spring, try this lighter tea cake as an afternoon treat instead of an evening dessert. By 6 p.m.—kapha hour—our digestion tends to slow down. For this reason, it's best to enjoy a light dinner and eat your sweets in small amounts in the daytime.

PREP: 10 minutes | COOK: 50 minutes | YIELD: 8 servings

DRY INGREDIENTS

1 cup finely ground cornmeal or polenta

1 cup spelt flour

1 cup coconut sugar

2 teaspoons baking powder

1 tablespoon, plus 1 teaspoon fennel seeds

½ teaspoon salt

WET INGREDIENTS

1 cup almond milk

¾ cup olive oil

3 tablespoons ground flax whisked into ½ cup water

1 tablespoon plus 1 teaspoon orange blossom water

Preheat the oven to 375°F. In a large bowl, combine the dry ingredients. In a separate bowl, combine the wet ingredients. Fold the wet ingredients into the dry, mixing together until fully combined.

Line a 9 x 5-inch loaf pan with parchment paper or grease with oil. Pour the batter evenly across the pan. Bake for 45–50 minutes, until golden outside and the batter is fully cooked inside. Use a toothpick to test if the center of the loaf is done. Remove from the oven and allow to cool before serving. Enjoy with your favorite cup of tea for an afternoon treat.

DOSHA NOTES

Ⓥ Enjoy as is.
Ⓟ Enjoy as is.

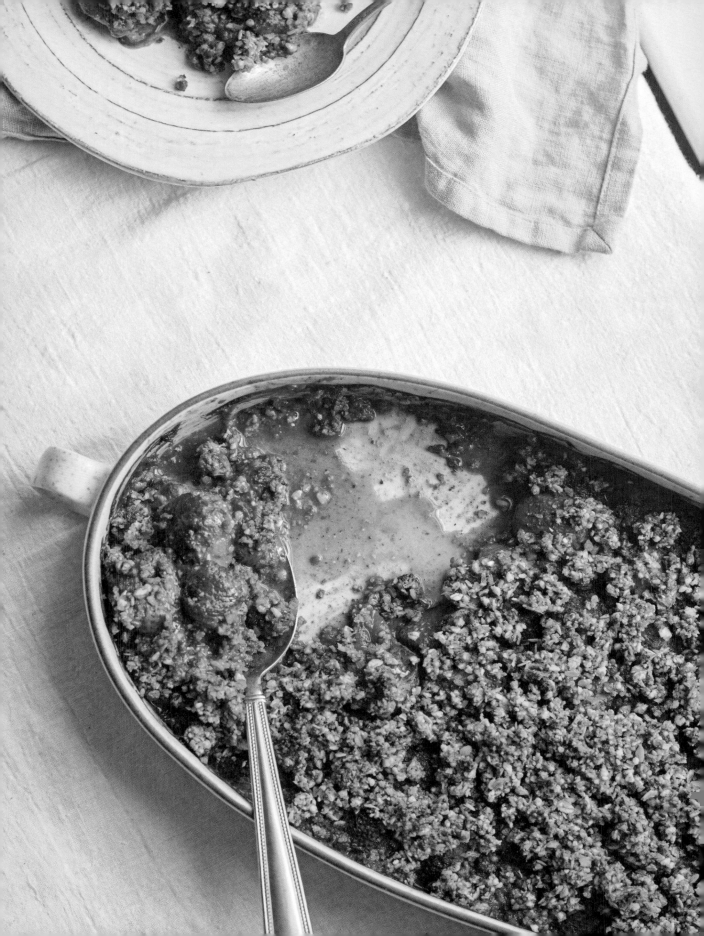

Strawberry Crisp

Berries are some of the lowest glycemic fruit. When cooked they can be combined with other foods and digested more easily than when raw. This crisp uses strawberries, digestive-promoting spices, and a small amount of coconut sugar for a low-glycemic sweet treat.

PREP: 15 minutes | COOK: 35 minutes | YIELD: 4–6 servings

TOPPING

1 cup whole raw almonds

½ cup organic rolled oats

4 tablespoons coconut sugar

2 tablespoons ghee or coconut oil

1 tablespoon lemon zest

1 tablespoon lemon juice

1 teaspoon ground cinnamon

1 teaspoon vanilla extract

½ teaspoon dried ginger

½ teaspoon ground turmeric

¼ teaspoon salt

FILLING

6 cups whole strawberries, stems removed

1 tablespoon vanilla extract

¼ teaspoon ground cardamom

For the topping: Preheat the oven to 400°F. In a food processor, add the almonds and pulse to break down into a roughly chopped pulp. Add the remaining ingredients and pulse a few times until combined. It will form a loose, crumbly mixture. Set aside while you prepare the filling.

For the filling: In a large mixing bowl, combine all ingredients and toss to mix. Spread the filling in an 8 x 8-inch baking pan. Layer the topping evenly over the strawberries. Bake for 35–45 minutes, until the berries are fully cooked down and gooey, and the topping becomes golden and crispy. Remove from the oven, allow to cool in the pan for 30 minutes, letting the flavors mature as it cools before serving.

Note: Fresh strawberries are preferred, but if using frozen, be sure to thaw and drain the excess liquid before using.

DOSHA NOTES

Ⓥ Serve with a spoonful of organic yogurt.

Ⓟ Omit ginger.

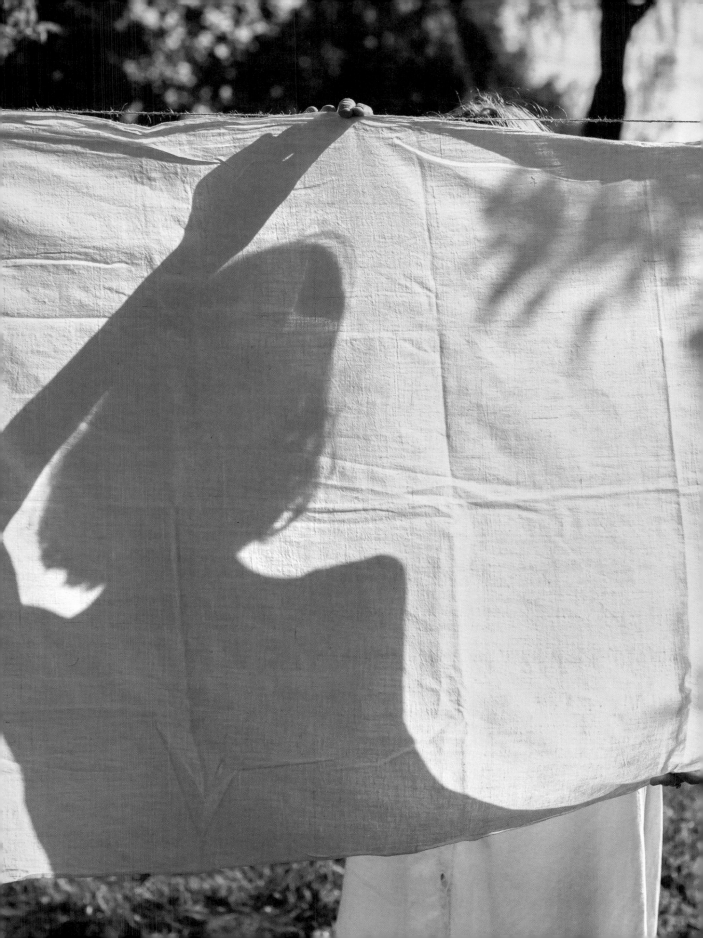

SUMMER

Long days. Juicy, ripe fruit dripping down sticky hands. Biting into summer.

Summer is pitta season. With the hot, sharp, and intense qualities of the summer months, we need to adopt a softness and an attitude of playfulness to find balance. Staying cool is the name of the game in our hot weather practice. When our surrounding environment heats us up, we look to our food, breath, and movement practices to balance pitta with soothing, calming, and cooling qualities. Your warm-weather kitchen is stocked with foods that are sweet, bitter, and astringent— think juicy stone fruit and melons, leafy greens, and sweet grains. With more activities in the sun and adventures stretching into longer days, vata also increases in summertime, which is why creating stability through daily routine is especially valuable this time of year. As you move through summer, try these soothing yoga and pranayama sequences, rituals that get you under the cool moonlight and enjoying the outdoors, and recipes that work with nature's juicy flavors.

Staying Balanced through Summer

EMPHASIZE

FOOD: Sweet, bitter, and astringent foods that are lightly cooked, raw, and simply spiced; cooling herbs and spices, juicy sweet fruit, fresh leafy greens, water-dense vegetables; ensure a consistent meal routine with light snacks as needed to stay fueled and hydrated.

BREATH: Soothing breathing that expels excess heat and calms the mind, such as Sitali, Nadi Shodhana, or Sama Vritti pranayama that focus on even, rhythmic inhalations and exhalations; lunar breathing through the left nostril.

MOVEMENT: Try steady, strengthening, vigorous, and heating asana with longer-held postures. If not yoga, ask yourself in what ways can you move your body that will bring joy and a sense of vibrancy to your day.

MEDITATION: Playful, engaging, and dynamic movement with a cooling breath and attitude; moon salutations and poses that support the small intestine, liver, and stomach, including twists, side bends, gentle backbends, and shoulderstands.

MINIMIZE

FOOD: Overly salted, spicy, oily and fried foods; pungent and excessively sour tastes; eggs; alcohol; black tea; coffee; fasting too long between meals.

BREATH: Breathing that is sharp or intense and builds internal heat, such as Kapalbhati, Bhastrika, and strong ujjayi breathing during asana.

MOVEMENT: Vigorous movement, especially in peak daytime hours (10 a.m.–2 p.m.) in direct sunlight; yoga or exercise in heated rooms; competitive attitude and environments.

Tips for Tending Your Inner Fire in Summer

The extra heat and activity of summertime can fan the flames of agni, try these simple tips for protecting your inner fire:

- Instead of chugging ice water, cool yourself down with infused waters. Add sliced cucumber, fresh mint, or a splash of rose water to your room-temperature water and sip throughout the day. Enjoy Rehydration Lemonade (page 158) if over-heated and dehydrated from too much time in the sun.

- Summer is the season of ripe, juicy fruit. Be sure to enjoy this alone in the morning as a simple breakfast or in the afternoon between meals as a refreshing snack. Combining raw fruit with dairy or a protein is a sure way to slow down digestion. Eat it alone or well cooked to increase digestibility.

- If you have vata- or kapha-type digestion, avoid overdoing it on the raw vegetables. Enjoy salad for lunch, when pitta is highest and supports digestion. Lightly braise, steam, or sauté vegetables for evening meals or when digestive fire is low.

- For fiery pitta-type digestion, make sure to keep a routine around eating. When you're out and about, pack a lunch and a light afternoon snack. Fasting too long between meals can create acid reflux and other pitta-associated belly troubles.

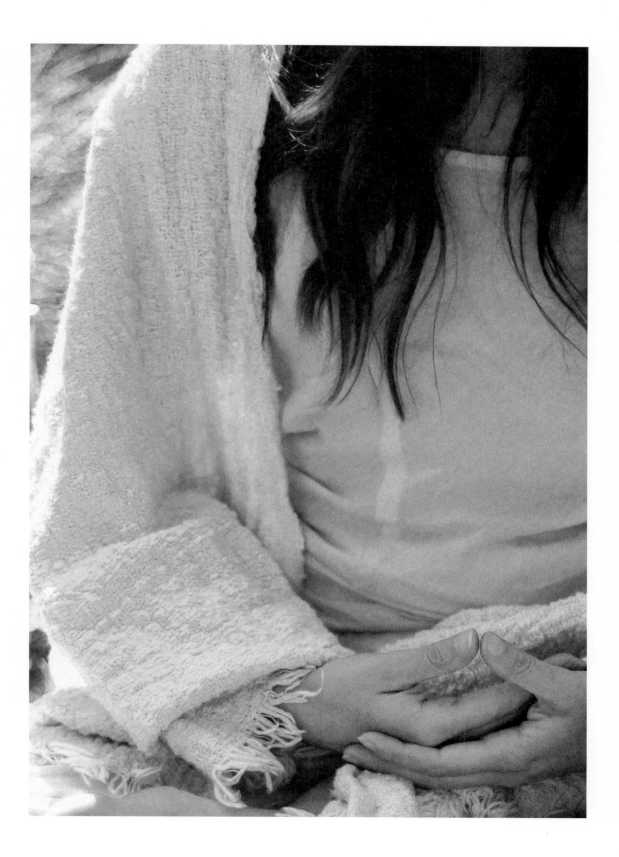

Summer Asana: *Soothing*

Perfectionism is the pesky quality of pitta that can rear its head especially in summertime. I bring this up in the summer asana section because play is a perfect practice for letting go of the controlling and constricting energy that can arise when pitta is high. Laugh at yourself and make fun of life a bit! Humility and playfulness are the antidotes to our inner critic.

This pitta-balancing sequence of gentle backbends, twists, and seated forward folds relieves built-up heat in the body. Try this sequence as it is, but don't be afraid to mix it up and get creative. Play around with fluidity between postures without trying to perfect the poses or match your breath perfectly with the movement. Keep your gaze soft, your breath fluid, and your mind at ease. Most importantly, don't be afraid to slow down and rest when needed. Remember, with increased pitta comes increased vata; this sequence aims to balance both. As you move through this practice, as yourself, "How can I use 10 percent less effort in each posture? Where can I breathe more humility and flexibility into my life?"

SUMMER PRACTICE TIPS

- Create a comfortable practice space with plenty of air circulation.

- Skip the heated rooms or placing your mat in direct sunlight to prevent overheating.

- Practice at a moderate pace and keep your intensity in check.

- Flow and move with ease and playfulness.

- Breath with a soft ujjayi. Exhale through your mouth occasionally to release built-up heat or tension. Even let out a few sighs and make audible noises when needed.

- Keep your jaw and shoulders relaxed and soften your gaze. It's easy to clench your jaw and upper-body muscles when overly focusing.

- Ditch any comparisons, self-criticism, or judgment.

DOSHA NOTES

Ⓥ Less is more if you're feeling depleted. Try this sequence slowly and with focused, steady breathing.

Ⓚ Incorporate stronger ujjayi breathing and longer holds in postures.

BALASANA (CHILD'S POSE)

Sit your hips back to your heels and lay your chest on your thighs. Place your forehead on the floor and draw your arms back by your feet with palms facing up. Hold for 10 breaths.

MODIFICATIONS

- Widen your knees and rest your chest between your legs, extend your arms forward.

- Place a cushion or folded blanket between your calves and thighs for knee support.

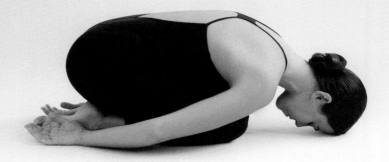

VIRASANA (HERO'S POSE) WITH NECK & SHOULDER ROLLS

Sit on your heels with your knees together. Rest your hands on your thighs with your palms facing down and relax your shoulders. Inhale, lengthen your tail bone toward the floor. Exhale, relax your chin to your chest. Hold for 1–2 breaths. Inhale, lift your head to neutral. Exhale, draw your right ear to your right shoulder. Inhale, lift your head to neutral. Exhale, draw your left ear to your left shoulder. Alternate sides 3–5 times.

MODIFICATIONS

- Sit on a block or place a cushion or folded blanket between your calves and thighs for knee support.

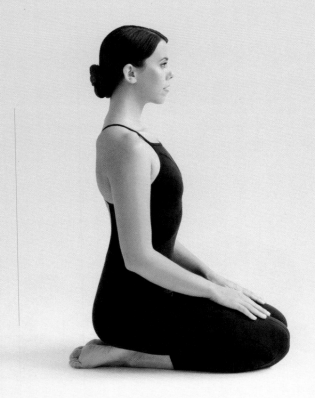

MARJARYASANA & BITILASANA (CAT & COW SEQUENCE)

Come to a tabletop position, with your fingers spread wide and your knees hip-width apart. Lengthen your spine long and draw your navel in to engage your abs. Inhale, lift your tailbone to the sky and arch your back, extend the crown of your head toward your hips, and squeeze your shoulder blades together. Exhale, press the ground away with straight arms, round your upper back, draw your chin to your chest, and point your tailbone toward the earth. Repeat for 1–2 minutes.

MODIFICATIONS

- Place a blanket beneath your knees for padding. For wrist sensitivities, form fists with your hands or come down onto your forearms.

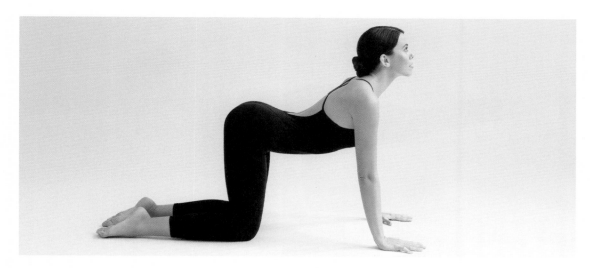

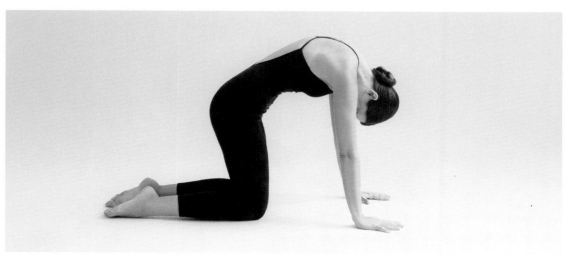

CHAKRAVAKASANA (SUNBIRD SEQUENCE)

Continue on your hands and knees. Inhale, extend your right leg behind you at hip height and your left arm forward at ear height. Flex your heel and point your toes toward the earth. Keep your pelvis level. Exhale, draw your elbow and knee into your chest, round your upper back. Inhale, extend your arm and leg back out. Reach your arm in opposition to lengthen your spine. Repeat 3–5 times on each side.

MODIFICATIONS

- Place a blanket beneath your knees for padding.

- For more stability, keep both hands on the ground while lifting each leg.

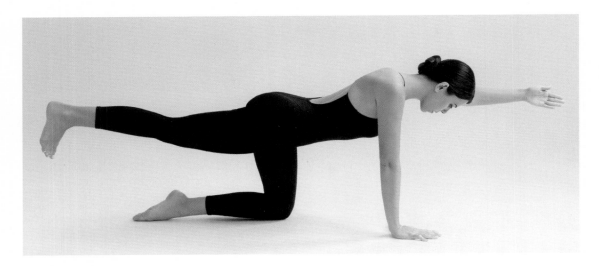

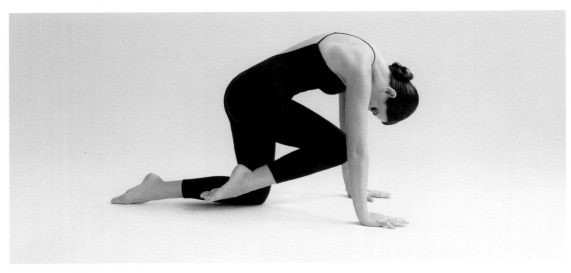

ANAHATASANA (MELTING HEART POSE)

Continue on your hands and knees. Keep your hips aligned over your knees, then walk your hands forward until your forehead meets the ground. Rest your chest on the ground. Hold for 3–5 breaths.

MODIFICATIONS

- Place a pillow or bolster below your chest for support.

- Try this standing at a wall, 2 feet away, with your arms stretched up the wall.

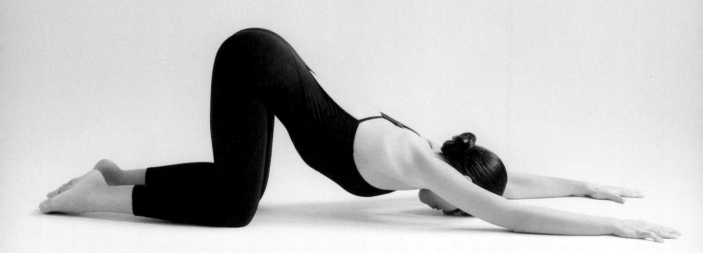

PASCHIMOTTANASANA (SEATED FORWARD BEND)

Sit upright with your legs extended straight in front of you. Flex your feet, pressing into the heels and balls of your feet to lengthen your legs. Inhale, sit tall. Exhale, bend at your hips to fold over your legs. Hold your ankles or wrap your hands around your feet. Hold for 3–5 breaths.

MODIFICATIONS

- Elevate your hips with a folded blanket. Use a strap or belt around your feet.

- Bend your knees if there is pain in your legs or low back.

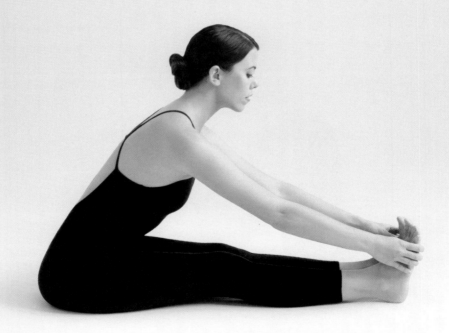

JANU SIRSASANA (SEATED HEAD-TO-KNEE POSE)

Sit upright with your legs extended straight in front of you. Bend your left knee to your chest and rotate your knee down to the ground. Firmly press your left foot to your right upper inner thigh. Inhale, sit tall. Exhale, hinge at your hips to fold over your legs, and hold either side of your right ankle or wrap your hands around your right foot. Hold for 5 breaths. Repeat on the other side.

MODIFICATIONS

* Elevate your hips with a folded blanket. Use a strap or belt around the feet.

* For knee sensitivities, place a rolled blanket or towel behind your extended knee.

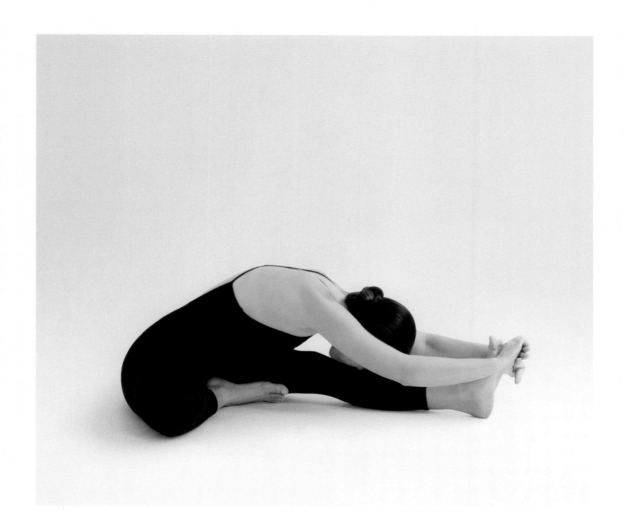

ARDHA MATSYENDRASANA (HALF FISH POSE)

Sit upright with your legs extended straight in front of you. Bend your right knee to your chest and place your right foot to the outside of your left knee. Bend your left knee and draw your left foot back by your hip. Inhale, reach your left arm to the sky and lengthen your spine. Exhale, twist toward your right leg and wrap your left arm around your thigh. Place your right arm behind your sacrum on the ground for support. Hold for 3–5 breaths. Slowly unwind and repeat on the other side.

MODIFICATIONS

- Extend and straighten one leg.

- Sit in a chair and take a gentle twist on both sides for a milder variation.

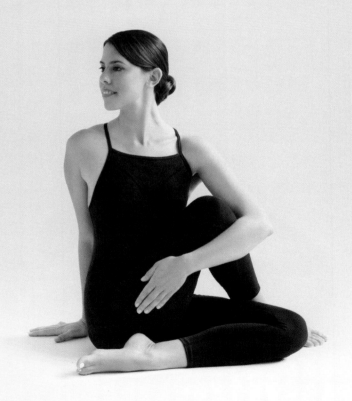

SUPTA PADANGUSTHASANA (RECLINED HAND-TO-BIG-TOE POSE)

Lie flat on your back with your legs extended long. Inhale, lift your right leg and catch your big toe with your right hand, wrapping your index and middle fingers around the toe. Keep your left leg straight on floor with your foot flexed. Hold for 3–5 breaths. Open your leg out to the right side, keeping both glutes on the ground and your hips level. Hold for 3–5 breaths. Draw your leg back to center and lower to the ground. Repeat on the other side.

MODIFICATIONS

- Use a strap or belt around your foot to relieve tight hamstrings.

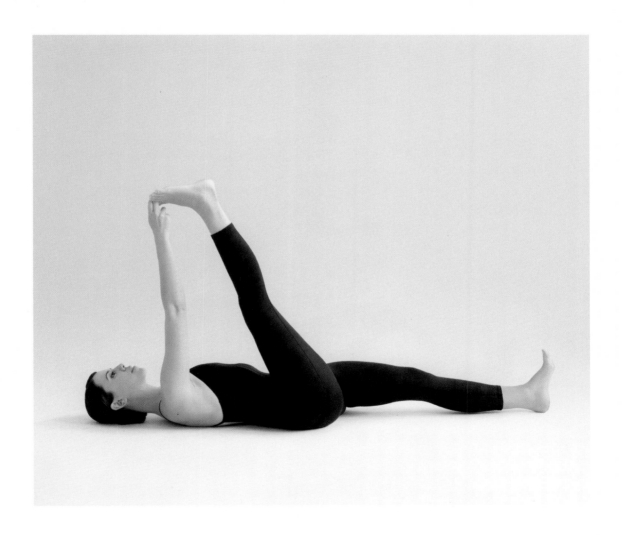

SUPTA BADDHA KONASANA (RECLINED BOUND ANGLE POSE)

Lie on your back on a rolled blanket or bolster in line with your spine. Bend your knees and place your feet on the ground. Open your legs and allow your knees to gently fall toward the ground. Draw the inner edges of your feet together. Rest your arms long by your sides with your palms facing up. Hold for 3–5 minutes.

MODIFICATIONS

- Sit on a blanket folded in half to elevate your hips and reduce low-back tension.

- Support your knees with pillows or blocks underneath each knee.

- Place a small pillow or folded blanket beneath your head for more elevation.

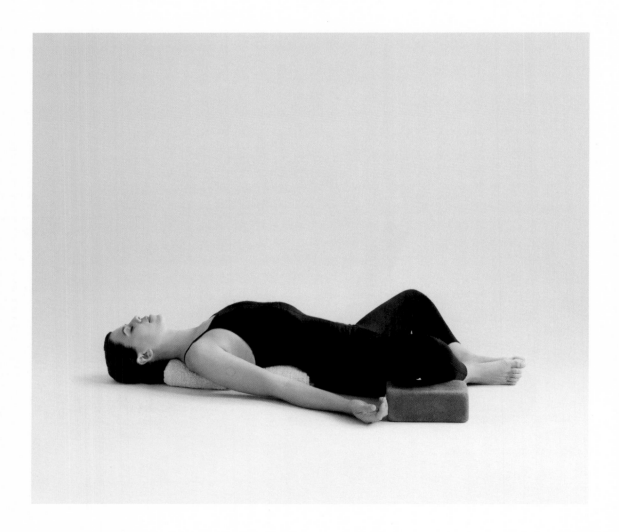

SAVASANA (CORPSE POSE)

The queen of all poses—do not skip this one! Lie on your back with your legs extended long and your arms resting by your sides, palms up. Close your eyes, exhale deeply, and relax every inch of your body. Relax any controlled effort to breathe. Rest in stillness for 7–10 minutes to complete your practice.

MODIFICATIONS
- Place a pillow or bolster behind your knees and use an eye pillow or cloth.

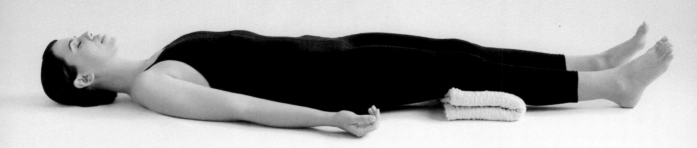

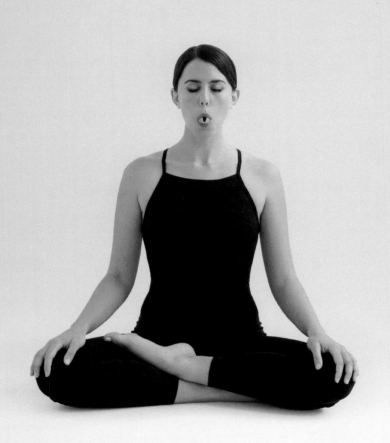

Summer Pranayama: *Sitali*

You know that point in summer when you're hot, agitated, a little short-tempered, and feeling stretched thin? This breathing practice is your hot-weather friend. *Sitali* helps reduce pitta's heating effects and balance the scattered energy of vata that comes from too much movement, bringing a cooling and calming quality to the body and mind. Practice this pranayama when you need to cool down.

HOW TO

Sitali moves the breath through the mouth instead of the nostrils. Inhaling through the mouth can quickly reduce body temperature, whereas more active nostril breathing (such as ujjayi) tends to heat the body. Because of this, it's best practiced in hot months or when you're feeling overheated. Skip this practice when you're cold, weak, or recovering from a chest cold or dampened lungs.

1   Sit in a comfortable position that supports your spine and hips. This can be done cross-legged on the floor or upright in a chair. However you choose to sit, make sure your hips are relaxed and your head, neck, and spine are aligned. Relax your shoulders, neck, and jaw. Soften your belly.

2   Open your mouth and extend your tongue just past your lips. Curl the edges of your tongue upward to create a tube or U shape with your tongue. If you can't do this (don't worry, it's a genetic thing!), simply make an O shape with your lips around your tongue, as if you were resting your mouth on a straw.

3   Inhale and breathe through your tongue, as if you were breathing through a straw, inhaling deeply into your abdomen and lower ribs. Notice the cooling sensation as you breathe in.

4   Draw your tongue back in and close your mouth, and hold the breath for a moment or two.

5   Slowly exhale through both nostrils.

6   Repeat 5–7 times, or up to 1 minute when needed.

PRACTICE NOTE

If you cannot curl your tongue in either tongue position in step 2, try folding back the tip of your tongue under your upper teeth and breathing through the sides of your folded tongue and mouth. This variation is sometimes called *sitkari*.

Summer Lunar Ritual: *Waxing Moon*

The period between the new and full moons is known as the waxing moon phase. This is a time of increasing energy and vitality, or *ojas*. Ojas is the subtle essence of kapha and the water element. Associated with the lunar cycles, it brings a juicy vitality with it. The waxing moon is a time when creativity naturally blossoms and we feel energized to start new projects. This waxing moon phase is a time of regeneration and gathering strength.

WOMEN'S LUNAR RITUALS

In a woman's cycle, the waxing moon phase aligns with the follicular phase before ovulation. It brings an increase of estrogen, a building hormone that lubricates, nourishes, and builds bodily tissues. After menstruation, kapha increases and your natural desire to create and engage with the outer world grows. In this time, oil massage, aromatherapy, dancing, and spending time outdoors in the moonlight all nurture an inner juiciness.

LUNAR BATHING

The moon has a particularly cooling effect on the body and mind and is cherished in summer as a rejuvenating antidote to the long days spent outdoors in the hot sun. The sun is associated with agni, but too much heat burns up our vital essence. The moon, associated with *soma* and the water element, has qualities that are soft, cooling, calming, and lubricating. Spending time under the moon reduces pitta and increases the nurturing effects of kapha.

In Vedic tradition, women would convene under the full moon to walk, tell stories, and bathe in the moonlight. As the moon waxes and grows brighter, this ritual invites you to get outside at night and spend time basking under the rays of the moon.

THE RITUAL

Shortly after the moon rises, take a blanket outside and spread it out under the moonlight. Take a seat or lie down. Spend 5–30 minutes in silence, gazing at the moon. Silence builds ojas. Sip the sweetness of a warm night under the cooling moon. It's as simple as that!

Summer Seasonal Ritual: *Solstice Celebration*

Summer solstice marks the longest day of the year and the height of pitta dosha for many climates. As the sun moves in a northerly direction, the period of increasing light between the winter and summer solstice is called *uttarayana*. This six-month cycle from winter to summer is characterized by the growth of new life and an outward, expansive energy. Solstice is a time to celebrate life and our own fullness. This seasonal ritual is all about connecting to that which makes us feel most vibrantly alive and sharing that with those we love.

HOSTING A GATHERING

Eating is a social act. It's a way we connect and share stories, telling tales of our adventures and what's inspiring us. We don't even have to speak the same language with our guests—food is the cross-cultural connector, the common tongue. This kind of nourishment comes not just from the types of food we eat but also the joy we experience while eating.

I love to host gatherings for this very reason. Cooking for others is my way of giving love, and in the process of giving, I receive so much in return. Eating together needn't be complicated. In a season where there's so much abundance, it's easy to stop by a farmers market and create a simple menu filled with the season's flavors. I suggest these menus. Mix and match greens, fill the tacos with summer squash or the summer rolls with herbs from your herb box.

GET OUTSIDE

There's a casual intimacy in meals shared outside. On a blanket spread on the grass or a long table under the trees, gather during the golden hour when the sun is low on the horizon and offers a cooler time to eat. As simple as this seems, spending time outside in cool fresh air is one of the recommended practices for soothing pitta in summer!

EAT WITH YOUR HANDS

In many cultures, eating with your hands is not only customary but also crucial for good health. The Ayurvedic map of the hand includes an element for each finger: thumb (ether), index (air), middle (fire), ring (water), pinkie (earth). When we eat with our hands, we unite the five elements and their associated senses. Poet Krishna Kant Shukla cleverly said that "eating with a knife and fork is like making love through an interpreter." By touching our food, we regain the sensual experience of nourishing ourselves. With that, we have a greater awareness and appreciation as a result.

SAVOR SLOWNESS

The French have a way of taking hours at a meal. They put their forks down between each bite, chew slowly and completely, and then spend several minutes engaged in conversation or contemplation before taking another bite. There's a presence that comes with moving slowly—presence with the food and with your company. Don't be shy to even take time in silence together. There's something profound about shared stillness in nature. Notice the positive effects this has on both your belly and your mood.

PICNIC MENU

- Hibiscus Sun Tea (page 156)

- Summer Rolls (page 174)

- Shaved Fennel Salad with Basil Vinaigrette (page 171)

- Rustic Fig Galette (page 187)

DINNER MENU

- Ginger Appetizers (page 64)

- Mint & Brahmi Tea (page 158)

- Coriander Beet Soup with Coconut-Dill Cream (page 168)

- Mung Bean Tacos (page 178)

- Digestive Lassi (page 65)

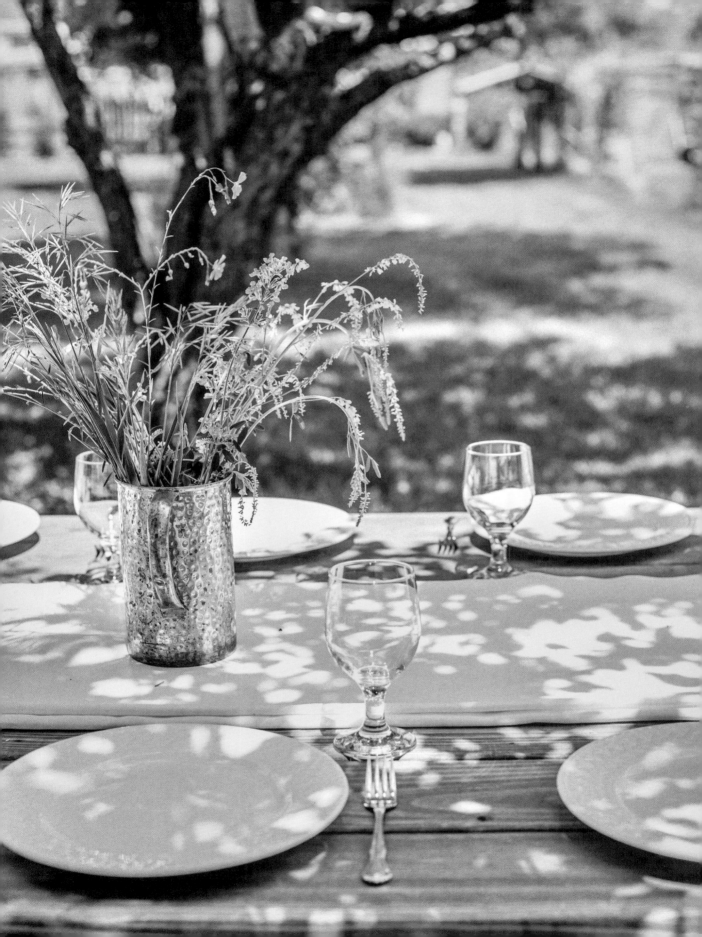

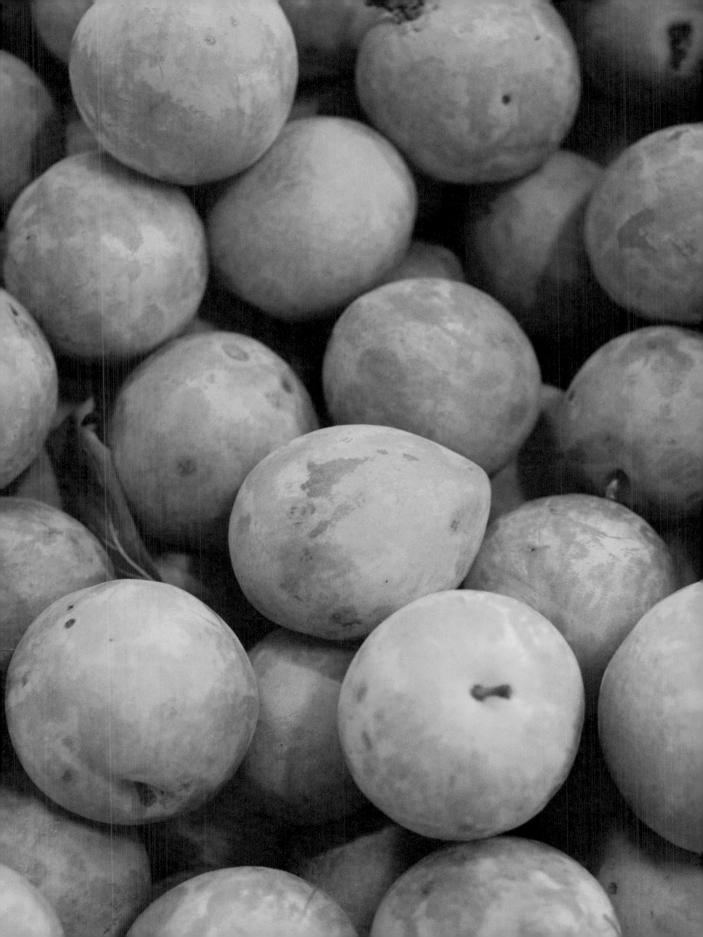

Summer Recipes

Hibiscus Sun Tea

Sweet, bitter, and astringent are the three tastes for soothing pitta. This simple summer sun tea contains all three and makes for a great midafternoon cooldown. Hibiscus is also a powerful blood tonic and can help reduce water retention.

PREP: 2 minutes | COOK: 4–6 hours | YIELD: 6 servings

½ cup dried hibiscus flowers

2 cinnamon sticks

7 cups filtered water

¼ cup lime juice

¼ cup raw honey

For garnish: lime wedges or fresh mint

In the morning, combine the hibiscus flowers and cinnamon sticks in a large 2-quart glass mason jar. Fill with 7 cups water. Seal with a lid and place outside in direct sunlight. Infuse for 4–5 hours, letting the heat from the sun steep the herbs. Watch as the color takes on a deep red hue as the hours go by. Once done, bring back to the kitchen to add the lime juice and raw honey. Seal with the lid again and shake until the honey is dissolved. Store in the fridge to cool down. Strain the pulp from the liquid when serving. Garnish with a lime wedge or sprig of fresh mint. Will keep for 2–3 days sealed in a jar in the fridge.

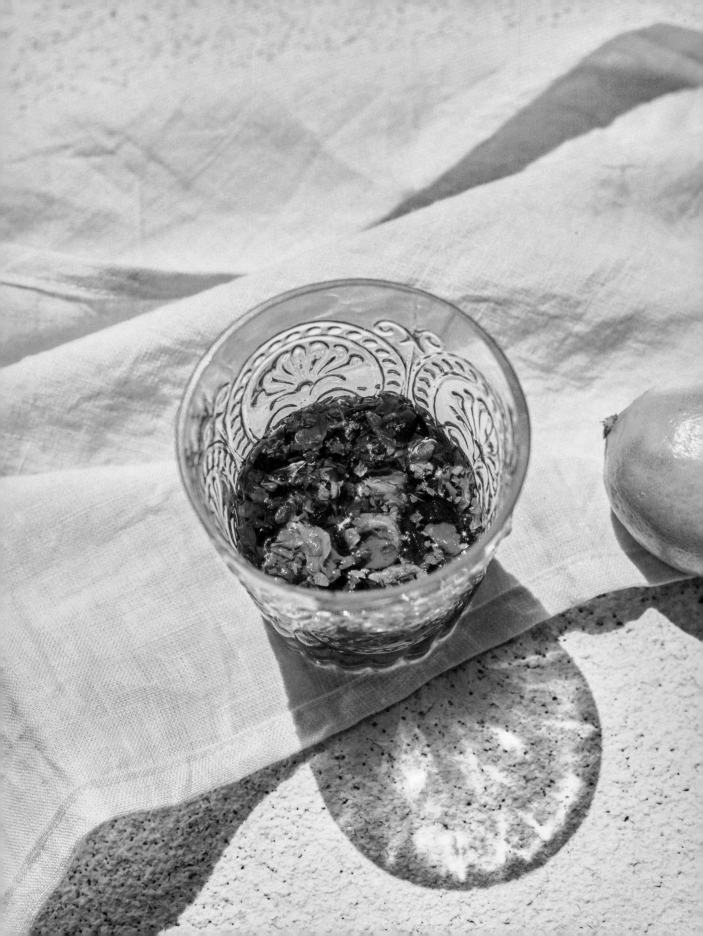

Mint & Brahmi Tea

Brahmi is a perennial that grows widely around the world and is often recognized by different names in different cultures. In India, it's known as "the herb of grace" for its soothing, sattvic qualities. Brahmi is one of the best herbs for balancing and rejuvenating pitta. Mentioned in the *Caraka Samhita* and *Sushruta Samhita* for promoting intelligence, longevity, and rejuvenation, this herb is recommended by practitioners in a variety of forms—from an herbal ghee to take internally to a decocted oil you can rub onto your head. Try adding it to this simple tea for a soothing summer drink.

PREP: 2 minutes | COOK: 10 minutes | YIELD: 2–4 servings

4 cups water

½ cup mint leaves (fresh or dry)

1 teaspoon dried brahmi

In a small pot, bring water to a boil. Once boiling, turn off heat and add the mint and brahmi. Cover with a lid and steep for 10 minutes. Strain the liquid and discard the pulp. Sip warm or store in a sealed jar in the fridge for a cool afternoon drink. Will keep for 2–3 days sealed in a jar in the fridge.

Rehydration Lemonade

Consider this recipe your Ayurvedic Gatorade, without the funky neon colors and artificial flavorings. Sip this hydrating drink when you might need an electrolyte boost—after asana, outdoor adventures, or time in the sun.

PREP: 5 minutes | COOK: 10 minutes | YIELD: 2–4 servings

4 cups warm water

½ cup lemon juice

2 tablespoons raw honey

½ teaspoon ground turmeric

¼ teaspoon mineral salt

Combine all ingredients in a large quart-sized mason jar. Seal with a lid and shake well to dissolve the honey and salt. Place in the fridge to chill before drinking. Will keep for 2–3 days sealed in a jar in the fridge.

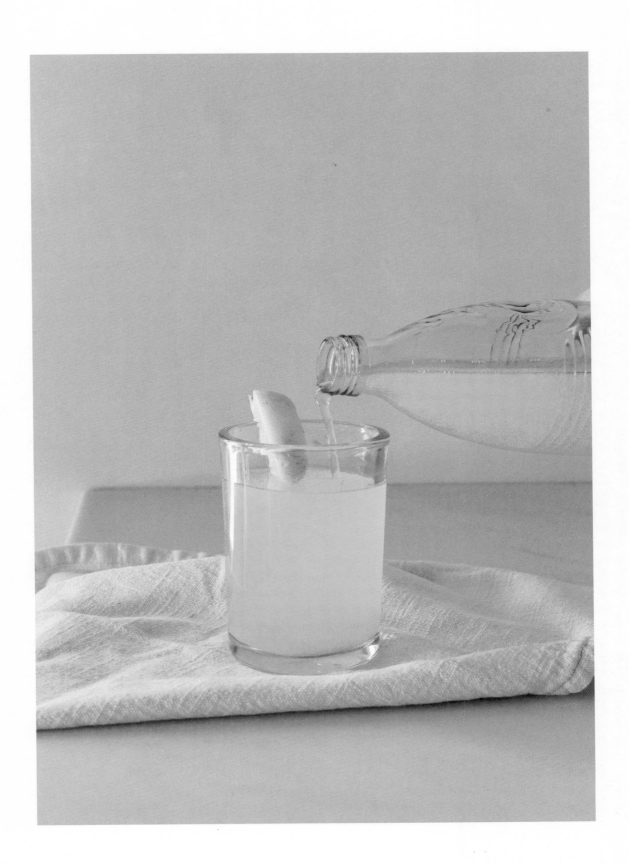

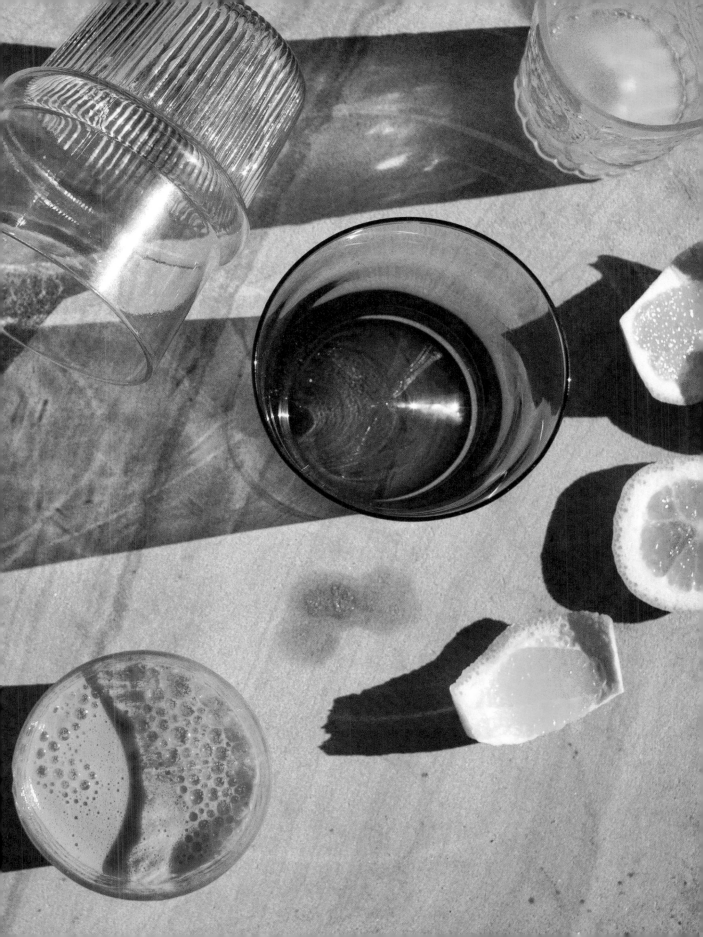

Summer Glow Juice

There's nothing more satiating than a thirst-quenching juice in summertime. This skin-boosting tonic loads you up with beta-carotene and vitamin A to protect the liver and purify the blood, balancing pitta along the way.

PREP: 5 minutes | COOK: 5 minutes | YIELD: 1–2 servings

4 carrots, scrubbed and trimmed

1 cucumber, peeled

1 orange, peeled

3 inches fresh turmeric root

Process all ingredients through a juicer. Pour into a glass and enjoy. This juice is best enjoyed right away.

Coconut Chia Breakfast Bowl

This easy chia porridge is my summer go-to when I know I have a busy morning ahead or need some nourishment that will hold well while traveling. Balanced with oats and creamy coconut milk, the sweet tastes of this bowl offer a soothing pitta-friendly breakfast. I like to make this recipe the night before a trip and store in a jar to take with me. It makes an easy camping breakfast or road-trip snack.

PREP: 5 minutes | COOK: 20 minutes | YIELD: 2–4 servings

COCONUT CHIA PORRIDGE

½ cup chia seeds

¼ cup rolled oats

¼ shredded unsweetened coconut

½ teaspoon ground cardamom

2 cups coconut or almond milk

2 tablespoons maple syrup

TOPPINGS

Sliced mango or fresh berries

Toasted coconut

Bee pollen

In a large bowl, combine the chia seeds, rolled oats, coconut, and cardamom. Add the coconut or almond milk and maple syrup and stir well. Allow to sit for 15–20 minutes, stirring a few times to prevent clumping. Spoon about 1 cup of the chia mixture into a bowl or jar and top with sliced mango or fresh berries, toasted coconut, and bee pollen. Store the porridge in an airtight container in the fridge for up to a day.

DOSHA NOTES

Ⓥ If stored in fridge, bring to room temperature before eating.

Ⓚ Reduce sweetener.

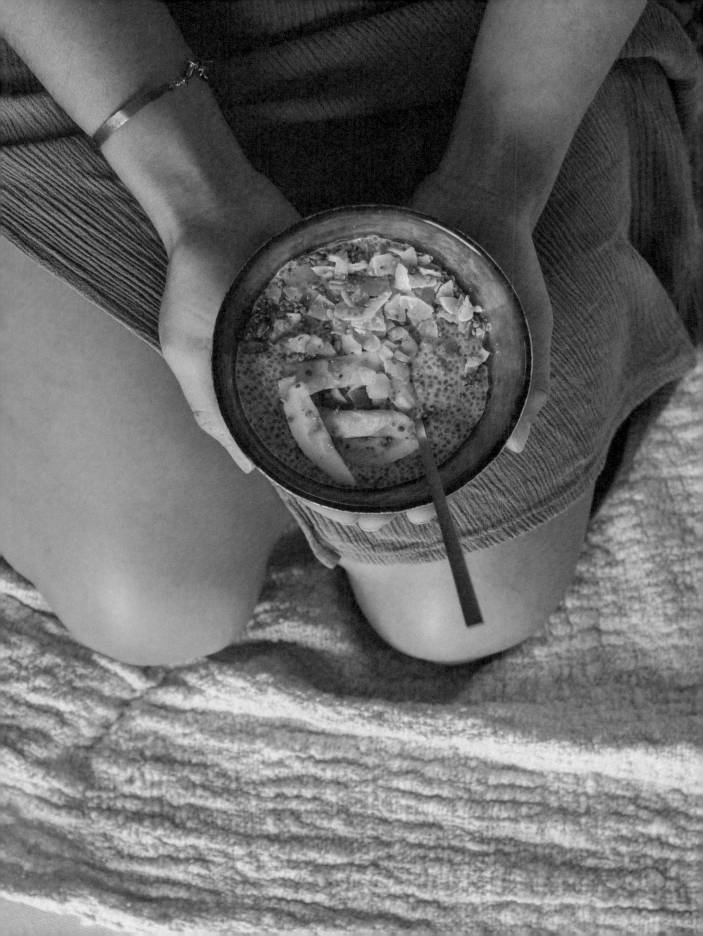

Zucchini & Herb Stuffed Paratha

Paratha is simply a stuffed chapati, made with sweet or savory ingredients. You can try chopped dates and walnuts, pumpkin, or sautéed spinach and potatoes, to name a few seasonal filling ideas. This summer breakfast paratha uses cooling zucchini and fresh savory herbs. Whole wheat is sweet and nourishing for pitta, making this a simple and satisfying option for a strong digestive fire. Admittedly, making paratha is not the easiest process at first. It may take a few tries to get your rhythm with rolling out the dough, but with persistence this can become a quick and easy breakfast standard.

PREP: 30 minutes | COOK: 10 minutes | YIELD: 2–4 servings

1 zucchini, grated

4 tablespoons fresh herbs (basil, oregano, parsley), finely chopped, plus more for serving

¼ teaspoon salt

Chapati dough (page 73)

1–2 tablespoons ghee or sunflower oil

Optional: 1 ounce goat cheese and/or poached egg

Squeeze grated zucchini to removed excess water, then place in a small mixing bowl. Add the chopped herbs and salt. Mix to combine. Set aside.

Preheat a well-seasoned skillet on medium-high heat. Form the chapati dough into 3-inch balls. On a well-floured surface, roll out each disk halfway, until you have thick disks about 3–4 inches wide. Place a spoonful of the grated zucchini and herb mixture in the center of each disk. Working with 1 disk at a time, fold the edges into the center and then use your hand to smooth out the folds of the dough. Take your rolling pin and roll out the paratha until it's ¼-inch thick. Flip over and roll the other side. You'll want to do this process fairly quickly to avoid the liquid from the zucchini making the dough too wet.

Put a dab of ghee onto the hot skillet and place the paratha on top. Cook for 90 seconds or until golden on each side. Repeat with the remaining paratha. Serve hot a sprinkle of fresh chopped herbs on top and goat cheese, if desired. For a heartier breakfast, serve with a poached egg.

DOSHA NOTES
(V) Finish with an extra dab of ghee on top.
(K) Try spelt flour or a gluten-free blend for a lighter chapati dough.

Sattvic Green Soup

Cooked cucumbers might seem unusual, but trust me here. This simple sattvic green soup is my standard for a hot summer day. It's both cooling for the body and calming for the mind. If you have an abundant summer garden, zucchini also works in place of cucumbers.

PREP: 5 minutes | COOK: 10 minutes | YIELD: 2–4 servings

1 teaspoon ghee or olive oil

1 teaspoon ground coriander

½ teaspoon ground fennel seeds

2 cucumbers, peeled, seeded, and chopped

2 cups packed spinach

1 avocado, peeled and pitted

½ bunch cilantro, plus some for garnish

1 tablespoons lime juice

¼ teaspoon salt

2½ cups filtered water

In a medium saucepan, heat the ghee and toast the spices for a minute. Add the cucumber and stir to coat. Sauté for 5–7 minutes, until tender. Remove from heat and allow to cool for a few minutes.

In a high-speed blender, add the spinach, avocado, cilantro, lemon juice, and salt. Add in the cooked cucumbers. Cover with water and blend until creamy. Taste and adjust seasonings as desired. If you like a thinner soup, add in another ½ cup water and blend again. Serve with a garnish of cilantro.

DOSHA NOTES

Ⓥ Serve warm.

Ⓚ Omit the oil.

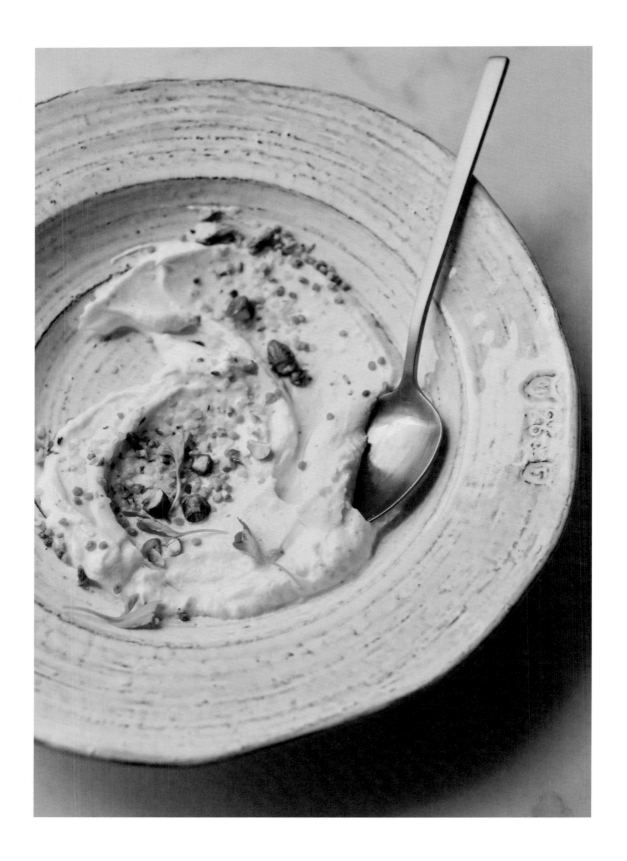

Saffron Orange Blossom Yogurt Bowl

Saffron is a powerful ally in summertime. Often used to soothe diseases caused by excess heat and to help purify the blood, this spice can be used in small amounts for its beneficial anti-inflammatory properties. One of my favorite flavor pairings is orange blossom water and saffron, a common combination you find in many Middle Eastern dishes. Try this spiced yogurt as a simple breakfast, but skip adding fruit to this bowl. Fruit is best eaten alone for better digestion.

PREP: 2 hours | COOK: 5 minutes | YIELD: 2 servings

YOGURT

2 cups organic plain coconut yogurt

2 teaspoons culinary orange blossom water or rose water

4–5 threads saffron

¼ teaspoon ground cardamom

TOPPINGS

Chopped pistachios

Hemp seeds

Dried rose petals

Put the yogurt in a wide cheesecloth-lined sieve set over a bowl. Cover, refrigerate, and let drain for 1–2 hours, until you have a thicker yogurt. You can speed the process a little by occasionally using a rubber spatula to lift and turn the yogurt.

When the yogurt is ready, mix the orange blossom water, saffron, and cardamom into the yogurt. If you're in a bind for time, the straining process can be skipped and the spices simply mixed into the yogurt. To serve, spoon 1 cup into a bowl and top with desired toppings.

DOSHA NOTES

Ⓥ Add a pinch of cinnamon.

Ⓚ Try pumpkin and flax seeds for toppings.

Fruit & Food Combining

Imagine your GI tract like a highway. You have fast-moving cars and slow-moving semitrucks. Proteins and fats are those heavy, slow-moving vehicles that take more time to digest, and fruit and carbohydrates are the quicker-moving vehicles. Fruit, which is sugar and water essentially, will break down quickly and move through your system freely when eaten alone. But when eaten with yogurt or protein, this combination can be like a traffic jam in your stomach and cause gas and bloating as a result. In summertime, all those juicy, ripe fruits are best eaten alone in the morning or as an afternoon snack several hours after lunch. Cooked fruit can be paired with grains and enjoyed in small quantities. Always trust your gut and check in with your digestive capacity when choosing a meal.

Coriander Beet Soup with Coconut-Dill Cream

A single ingredient prepared in different ways can have a variety of effects on the doshas. Beets, for example, can aggravate pitta when eaten raw but pacify it when cooked. Cooked beets have a sweeter taste, which calms pitta's fiery nature, nourishing the liver and cooling the blood. A cooling coconut-dill cream completes this creamy summer beet soup.

PREP: 10 minutes | COOK: 40 minutes | YIELD: 4 servings

CORIANDER BEET SOUP

2 tablespoons olive oil

2 teaspoons ground coriander

5 medium beets, peeled, trimmed, and cut into 1-inch cubes (about 5 cups)

5–6 cups water

1 teaspoon salt

1 tablespoon lemon juice

COCONUT-DILL CREAM

One 13.5 ounce can full-fat unsweetened coconut milk (½ cup coconut cream)

2 tablespoons fresh dill, finely chopped

¼ teaspoon salt

1 teaspoon lemon juice

In a large soup pot, heat the oil on medium heat. Add the coriander and beets. Cover with a lid and cook for 5 minutes, steaming the beets in their own moisture. Stir occasionally to prevent burning. Add the water and salt. Bring to a boil. Cover with a lid and reduce to medium heat and simmer for 45 minutes, until the beets are soft. Remove from heat and add the lemon juice. Transfer to a blender and puree. Work in batches as needed until all the soup is creamy. Serve warm or chilled with a dollop of coconut-dill cream on top.

For the cream: Place the can of coconut milk in the refrigerator for 30 minutes to chill. Scoop the cream off the top of the can. Combine in a bowl with 2 tablespoons coconut milk. Stir in the dill, salt, and lemon juice. Taste and adjust seasonings as desired.

DOSHA NOTES
Ⓥ Serve warm.
Ⓚ Reduce salt.

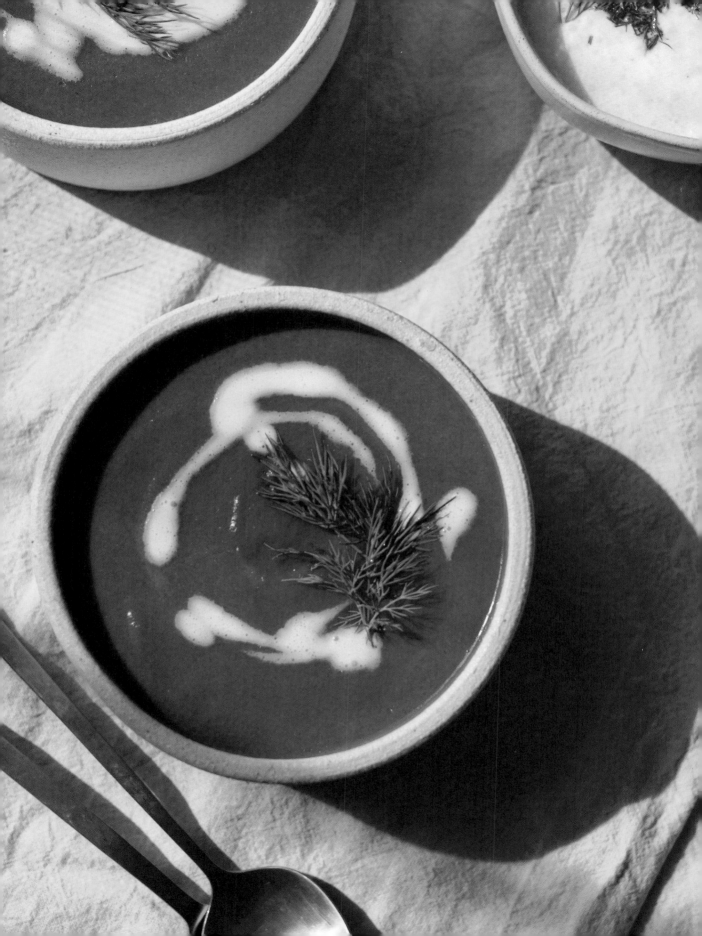

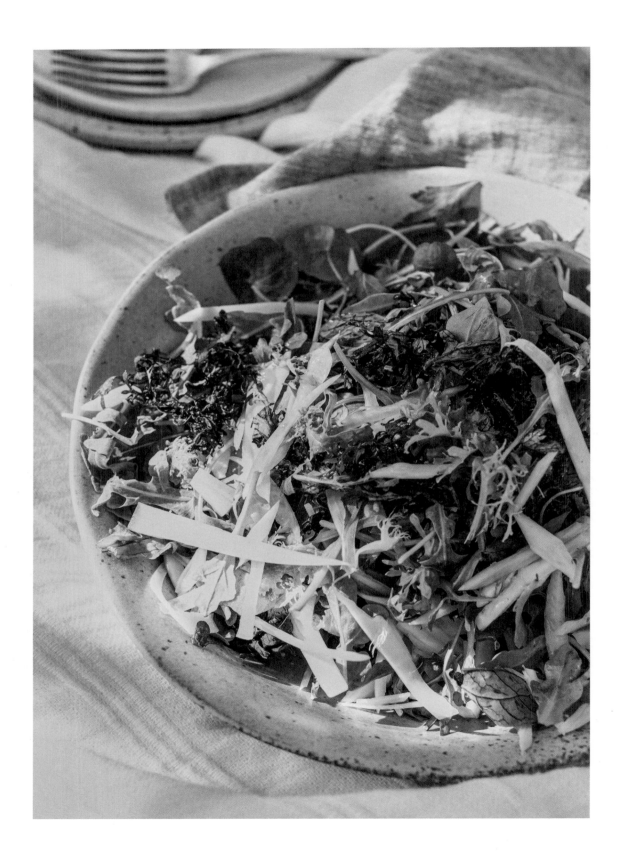

Shaved Fennel Salad with Basil Vinaigrette

I love a good salad with texture and rich flavors. Instead of your basic mixed greens, this chopped summer salad uses shaved fennel bulb and seeds for an added crunch. All parts of the fennel plant—seeds, bulb, and frond—are supportive for pitta. The fennel and fresh herbs in this recipe are slightly sweet and cooling. Enjoy this fresh herb salad at lunchtime when the sun is high and hot.

PREP: 15 minutes | COOK: 5 minutes | YIELD: 4–6 servings

SALAD

2 cups fresh greens (arugula, spinach, mesclun)

2 fennel bulbs, trimmed, quartered, and shaved thinly

¼ cup chopped basil

¼ cup chopped parsley

¼ cup chopped mint

½ cup pumpkin seeds

¼ cup hemp seeds

VINAIGRETTE

¼ cup olive oil

¼ cup flax oil

¼ cup lemon juice

1 tablespoon raw honey or maple syrup

2 tablespoons lemon zest

Salt and pepper, to taste

2 tablespoons basil, finely chopped

Combine all ingredients in a large bowl. Toss with vinaigrette before serving.

For the vinaigrette: In a small bowl, whisk together the oils, lemon juice and zest, and honey. Add the salt and pepper to taste, then fold in the basil. Store in a sealed jar in the fridge for up to 3 days until ready to serve. If cold, allow to come to room temperature and shake well before serving.

DOSHA NOTES

(V) Skip if digestive fire is weak.

(K) Use raw honey instead of maple in vinaigrette.

Crispy Okra

I first learned this recipe in South India from a beautiful woman who cooked for all the yoga students. She called this recipe *bhindi masala*. *Bhindi* is the Sanskrit word for okra. It has sweet and cooling properties beneficial for pitta, along with numerous medicinal benefits for all three doshas. It lubricates joints, relieves inflammation, protects the liver and kidneys by binding with toxins in the blood, and supports digestion as a prebiotic. Its slimy, mucilaginous qualities also lubricate the colon for healthy elimination. You'll find okra in season from July to September. A note on the spices here: Mango powder is her special add-in for this recipe, it's commonly found in Indian markets as amchoor powder, but this may be one spice you need to special order online. Substitute with a curry powder blend if you can't find mango powder or omit altogether, the okra still tastes great with this or without.

PREP: 15 minutes | COOK: 20 minutes | YIELD: 2–4 servings

1 teaspoon ground coriander

1 teaspoon ground cumin

1 teaspoon ground turmeric

¼ teaspoon salt

Optional: ½ teaspoon mango (amchoor) powder

30 whole okra

2 tablespoons sunflower oil or ghee

Lime juice, for serving

In a small bowl, combine the spices and salt. Wash and trim off the tops of the okra. Pat dry to remove any excess moisture and prevent oil splatter in the hot pan. Slit each okra lengthwise to create a pocket where the spices will be stuffed into. With a spoon, stuff each okra with about ¼ teaspoon of the spice blend. Set aside.

Heat a large skillet with oil on medium-high heat. Arrange the okra on the pan and fry for 2–3 minutes on each side. Turn the okra a few times to cook on all sides, cooking until tender on the inside and crispy on the outside. Transfer to a plate and squeeze a bit of fresh lime juice over top. Serve hot.

DOSHA NOTES

(P) Omit the mango powder if overheated.

(K) Use sunflower oil for frying

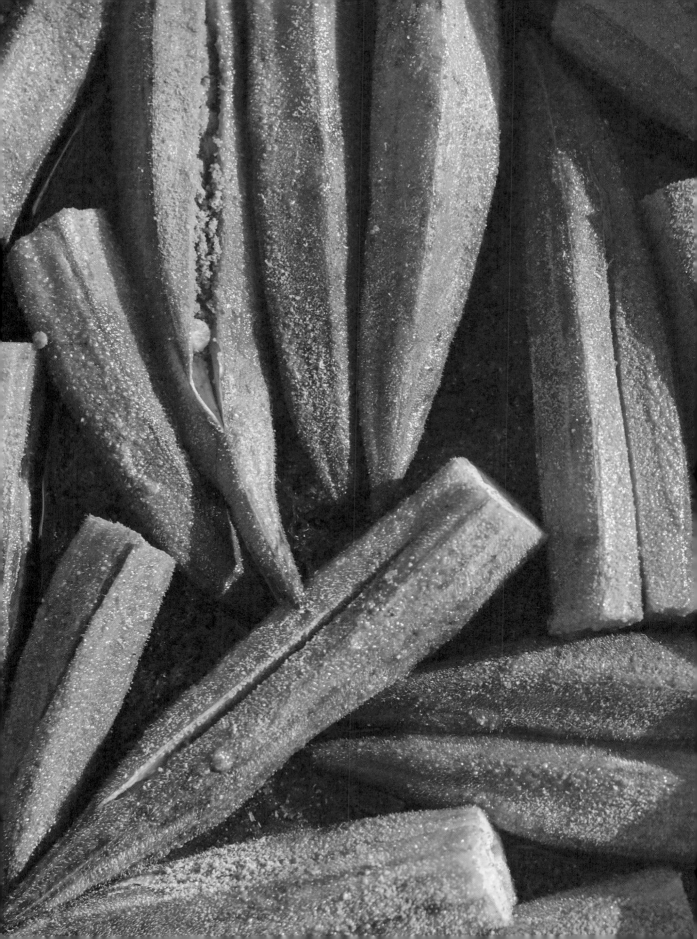

Summer Rolls

In the peak of summer, a hot meal is sometimes the last thing I want for lunch. These easy hand rolls are a great way to get out of the salad rut while still eating something light and refreshing. If making these in advance, keep them wrapped in a moist paper towel to prevent the rice wrappers from drying out and cracking.

PREP: 30 minutes | COOK: 20 minutes | YIELD: 4 servings

TURMERIC TOFU

8 ounces organic extra-firm tofu, sliced into ½-inch-thick slabs

2 tablespoons tamari

1½ tablespoons toasted sesame oil or sunflower oil

1 tablespoon lime juice

1 teaspoon ground turmeric

½ teaspoon ground coriander

ALMOND DIPPING SAUCE

½ cup almond butter

1½ tablespoons rice vinegar

1 tablespoon toasted sesame oil

1 tablespoon tamari

1-inch piece fresh ginger, roughly chopped

1 teaspoon maple syrup

1 tablespoon lime juice

½ cup water

Preheat the oven to 425°F. Gently arrange the tofu slices onto a paper towel and lay another over top. Press gently to absorb excess water. In a small bowl, whisk together the tamari, oil, lime juice, turmeric, and coriander. Arrange the tofu slices in a deep baking dish and pour the marinade on top. Allow to marinate for 10 minutes while the oven heats up. Bake for 20–25 minutes, until slightly firm and golden. Remove from oven and set aside to cool before wrapping.

For the sauce: Combine all ingredients in a blender. Puree until creamy. Add more water for a creamy but not overly thick consistency. Store in an airtight jar in the fridge until ready to use or for up 3 days.

SUMMER ROLLS

4 sheets rice paper

1 cucumber, peeled, deseeded, and julienned

1 avocado, peeled, pitted, and sliced

½ cup cilantro, roughly chopped

¼ cup mint, stems removed and roughly chopped

½ cup microgreens or sprouts

Prepare all the veggies and organize your rolling station. You want to have everything ready to grab when rolling the rice papers. Lay out a cutting board slightly damp with water to roll on, and place a wide bowl of hot water next to it. To soften the rice wrappers, dunk them into the bowl of hot water for 3–4 seconds and then remove. Avoid leaving them in the water for too long as they tear easily when they become too soft. Spread a wrapper across the cutting board and layer the veggies and tofu onto the center of the wrapper. Fold the sides in and then neatly roll. Repeat until done with your desired amount. Serve with dipping sauce.

Rolls are best eaten right away but can be stored for later in the day by wrapping them individually in moist paper towels to retain their moisture and freshness. The rice wrappers will crack if they become too dry. Store wrapped in the fridge until ready to serve.

Quinoa & White Bean Cakes with Avocado Dipping Sauce

These hearty quinoa and white bean cakes are packed with bitter greens and supporting spices. Enjoy these over greens or layered between a bun as a veggie burger. I like to pair this dish with Crispy Okra for a burger and fries feel.

PREP: 20 minutes | COOK: 20 minutes | YIELD: 6 servings

QUINOA & WHITE BEAN CAKES

1 tablespoon ghee or olive oil

6 chard leaves, finely chopped

2 cups white beans (fresh cooked or canned)

1½ cups cooked quinoa

¼ cup quinoa flour (chickpea or oat flour also works well), plus 2 tablespoons

3 tablespoons ground flax

2 tablespoons tamari

2 tablespoons lime juice

2 tablespoons finely chopped fresh basil

1 teaspoon ground cumin

½ teaspoon ground coriander

½ teaspoon ground fenugreek

½ teaspoon salt

Optional: Crispy Okra (page 180) or fresh greens, for serving

In a skillet, heat the oil on medium-high and add the chard. Sauté until cooked down, about a minute. Remove from heat and set aside. In a large bowl, mash the beans with a fork until they turn into a chunky paste. Add the sautéed chard, cooked quinoa, and remaining ingredients. Mix until well combined. With wet hands, form small patties about 3 inches wide and ¾-inch thick. If too wet, place the patties on a floured surface and coat each side with a little flour.

Heat a skillet with oil on medium heat and fry the patties on both sides until they are crispy and golden, about 2–3 minutes per side or longer. Serve warm with the dipping sauce (at right) over fresh greens or with a side of crispy okra.

AVOCADO DIPPING SAUCE

1 ripe avocado, peeled and pitted

¼ cup plain whole milk yogurt or yogurt of choice

½ bunch cilantro, roughly chopped

2 tablespoons lime juice

4 tablespoons water

½ teaspoon ground coriander

¼ teaspoon salt

For the sauce: Combine all ingredients in a blender and puree until creamy. Taste and adjust flavorings as desired. Transfer to a jar and store in the fridge for up to 1 day until ready to serve.

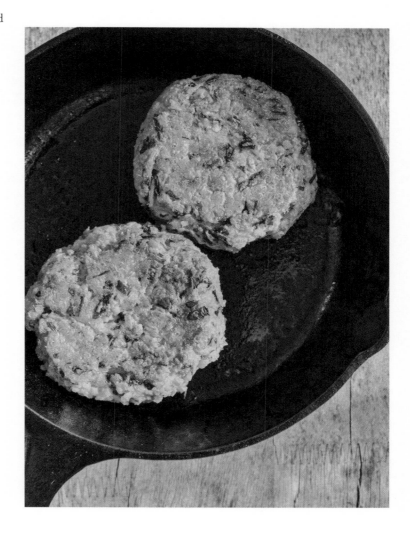

Mung Bean Tacos

In vegetarian cooking, sometimes you'll find overuse of soy products and textured vegetable protein (TVP) as a way to substitute animal proteins in meat-centered dishes—tacos being one of them. I've never been a big fan of these mock meat products, and I tend to steer clear of them altogether. I believe you can make a flavorful and balanced meal featuring simple ingredients as they are, no need for pretending. The versatile mung bean is the feature of this dish. When cooked down with molasses and spices, mung beans have a rich taste and texture that stands up to your standard taco filling. Try this with a chapati as a tortilla for this Ayurveda-inspired summer taco.

PREP: 20 minutes | COOK: 1 hour | YIELD: 4 servings

SAVORY MUNG BEANS

1 cup whole mung beans, soaked overnight

2 tablespoons ghee or olive oil

2 tablespoons coriander seeds

1 tablespoon cumin seeds

1 teaspoon fennel seeds

1 teaspoon ground fenugreek

1 tablespoon finely minced or grated fresh ginger

¼ teaspoon asafetida

2 tablespoons molasses

4 cups water

1 teaspoon salt

CHAPATI TORTILLAS
(page 73)

After soaking the beans overnight, drain and rinse well. Set aside.

In a large saucepan, heat the oil and add the spices, ginger, and asafetida to the pot. Stir frequently on medium heat until aromatic. Stir in the mung beans. Next, add the molasses and stir until well coated. Add the water and salt, cover, and reduce to a gentle simmer and cook until tender, about 35–40 minutes. You may need to add more water and cook longer. When the mung beans are slightly tender but not mushy, remove from heat and season with salt and pepper. Store or set aside until ready to use.

Prepare the Chapati dough while the mung beans are cooking. Once the mung beans are done, make the chapatis. Keep warm in a tortilla warmer or a pie dish lined with a tea towel. Serve hot.

continued

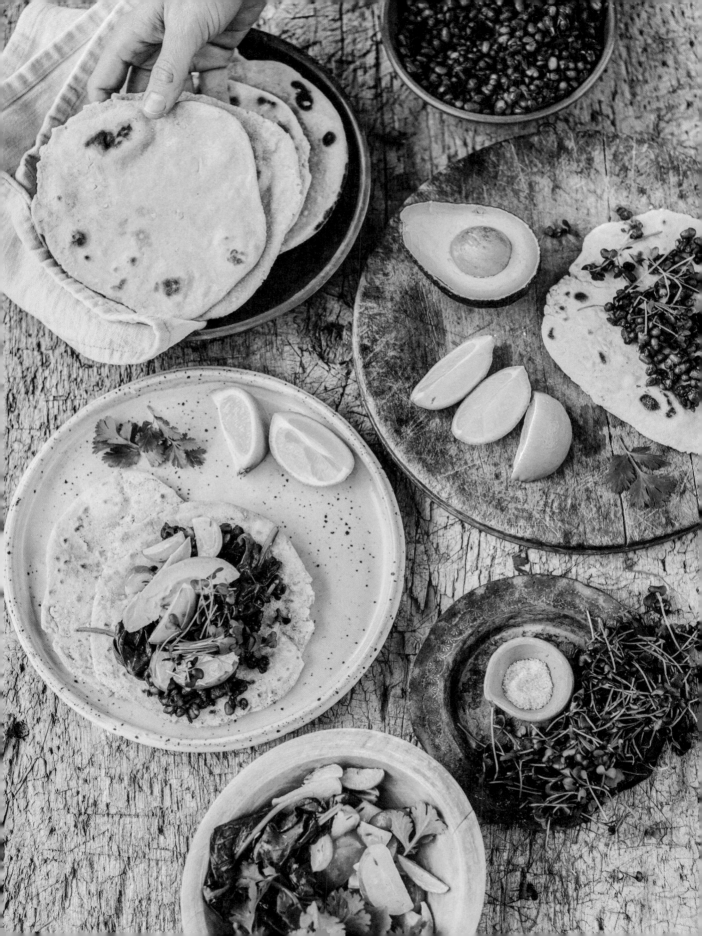

VEGGIES & GREENS

1 tablespoon ghee or olive oil

6 radishes (French breakfast, red/mixed color radishes), sliced into ¼-inch rounds

2 cups spinach

½ bunch cilantro, chopped

Squeeze of lime juice

Pinch of salt

TO ASSEMBLE

1 whole avocado, peeled, pitted, and sliced

¼ cup cilantro, roughly chopped

1 lime, quartered

For the veggies: In a medium saucepan, heat the oil on medium heat and add the radishes. Cover and cook until tender, about 7–10 minutes. Add spinach and cilantro and sauté the greens another minute until they are lightly steamed but not overcooked. This is a quick process. Add a squeeze of lime juice and season with salt. Serve hot.

When ready to serve, layer the mung beans and veggies onto a warm chapati and top with sliced avocado, cilantro, and a lime wedge.

DOSHA NOTES

Ⓥ Enjoy with extra avocado.

Ⓚ Serve with corn tortillas instead of chapati.

Chapati Pizza with Slow-Roasted Fennel, Squash & Parsley–Pumpkin Seed Pesto

In summer, I like to host what I call BYOP Night—Build Your Own Pizza. It entails making a series of mini crusts from chapati dough and friends bringing along the toppings. Together, we mix and match our own personal pizzas with the lineup of sauces and veggies. This pesto pizza with roasted fennel and butternut squash is now our favorite summer combo and a great pitta-friendly pizza.

PREP: 20 minutes | COOK: 50 minutes | YIELD: 6 servings

CHAPATI CRUST
(page 73)

PUMPKIN SEED PESTO
1 cup pumpkin seeds

1 cup tightly packed flat-leaf parsley

1 cup tightly packed arugula, plus fresh leaves for serving

1 cup tightly packed spinach

Optional: 1 small garlic clove

2 tablespoons lemon juice

½ teaspoon salt

½ cup olive oil

ROASTED BUTTERNUT SQUASH

1 small butternut squash, peeled, seeded, quartered, and thinly sliced

1 tablespoon olive oil

⅛ teaspoon salt

For the crust, follow the instructions for making Chapati. Let the dough sit while preparing the remaining components of the pizza. When ready, you can make one large chapati crust if you have a large enough skillet, or several smaller chapati crusts for a personal pizza option. Cast-iron works best for preparing this crust.

For the pesto: In a food processor or high-speed blender, pulse pumpkin seeds into a rough pulp. Add the parsley, arugula, and spinach and blend until broken down into a fine pulp. Then add the garlic (if using), lemon juice, and salt. Blend again until well incorporated. Add in the olive oil and pulse again to combine. Taste and adjust seasonings as desired. Store in a jar in the fridge for up to 3 days until ready to use.

For the squash: Preheat the oven to 400°F. Arrange the squash slices across a baking sheet, toss with olive oil and salt. Roast until tender, about 20 minutes. Remove from the oven and set aside.

continued

ROASTED FENNEL

1 fennel bulb, trimmed, halved vertically, and thinly sliced

1 tablespoon olive oil

⅛ teaspoon salt

While the squash is roasting, prepare the fennel. Spread fennel slices across a baking sheet, toss with olive oil and salt. Roast for 15 minutes, stirring occasionally to prevent sticking or burning. Reduce heat to 300°F and cook for another 20–30 minutes, until tender and caramelized. Remove from the oven. Leave the oven on while assembling the pizza.

To assemble: spread a thick layer of pesto on top of the chapati crust, then arrange the butternut squash and fennel on top. Place back in the hot oven to bake for 7–10 minutes. Remove from oven and finish with a couple of fresh arugula leaves.

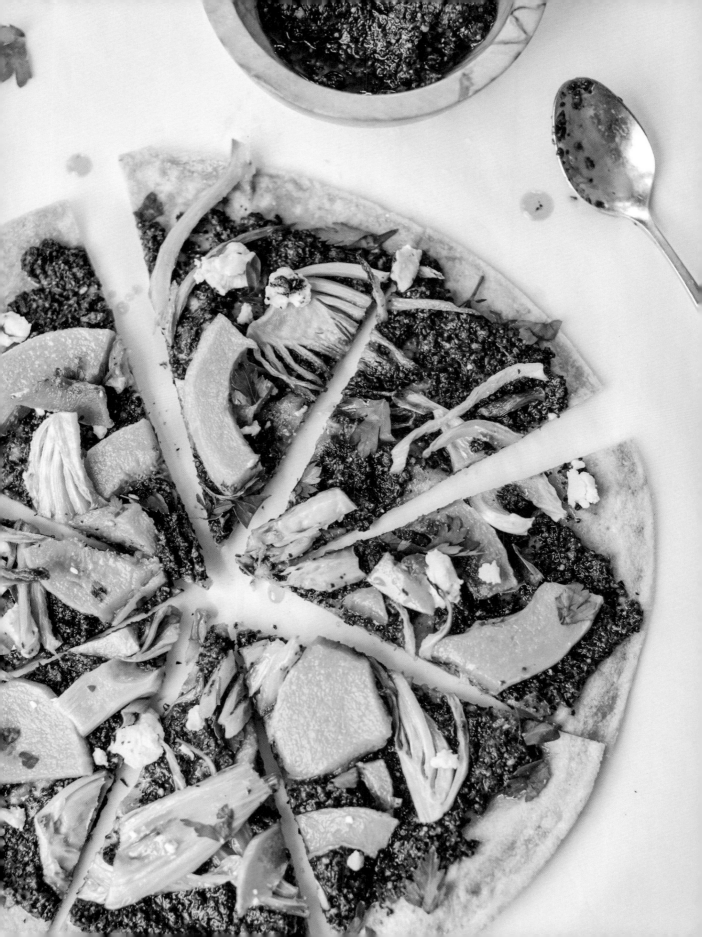

Creamy Coconut Curry Bowl

This sattvic summer curry bowl uses creamy coconut, kaffir lime, and fresh green vegetables as a cooling variation of a spicier winter favorite. Kaffir lime leaf is native to Southeast Asia and often used in Thai-style green curries. As it can be difficult to find in your regular grocery store, I've added extra lime zest and juice into this recipe to boost the flavor of this curry in lieu of the lime leaf. Serve this over coconut basmati rice and top with an extra handful of cilantro. For a protein boost, add cubed tofu to the curry toward the end of cooking.

PREP: 15 minutes | COOK: 30 minutes | YIELD: 4 servings

2 tablespoons coconut oil

2 tablespoons curry powder

1 tablespoon ground coriander

½ teaspoon ground fenugreek

1 teaspoon ground turmeric

1 teaspoon cumin seeds

1 small head broccoli or romanesco, cut into small florets

1 zucchini, trimmed and cut into ¼-inch-thick matchsticks

20 snap peas, trimmed and cut diagonally into ½-inch slices

Two 13.5-ounce cans unsweetened coconut milk

2 cups water

1½ teaspoons salt

2 cups chopped greens (chard, kale, collards)

1 bunch cilantro, roughly chopped, plus more for garnish

2–3 tablespoons lime juice

2 tablespoons lime zest

Optional: 4 fresh kaffir lime leaves

Lime wedges, for garnish

In a large pot, heat the oil on medium heat. Add the dry spices and heat for a moment until fragrant, stirring to prevent burning. Add the broccoli first, with a splash of water to steam for 1–2 minutes. Add the zucchini and peas, stir to coat with the spices. Add the coconut milk, water, salt, and kaffir lime leaves, if using. Bring to a simmer and cover with a lid. Cook for 15 minutes, until vegetables are tender. Add the spinach and cilantro, cook for another 10 minutes. Add the lime juice and zest at the end. Taste and adjust seasonings as needed. Serve hot over coconut basmati rice with a garnish of cilantro and lime wedge.

COCONUT BASMATI RICE

1½ cups water

1 cup white basmati rice

¼ cup organic shredded
unsweetened coconut

¼ teaspoon salt

For the rice: In a small pot, bring the water to a boil over high heat. Add the rice, coconut, and salt. Once the mixture returns to a boil, turn the heat down to low and cover with a lid. Cook for 18–20 minutes. Uncover and continue to cook for 5 minutes. Fluff with a fork and serve hot.

DOSHA NOTES

Ⓥ Add 1 tablespoon minced fresh ginger to the spice mix.

Ⓚ Use untoasted sesame oil instead of coconut oil.

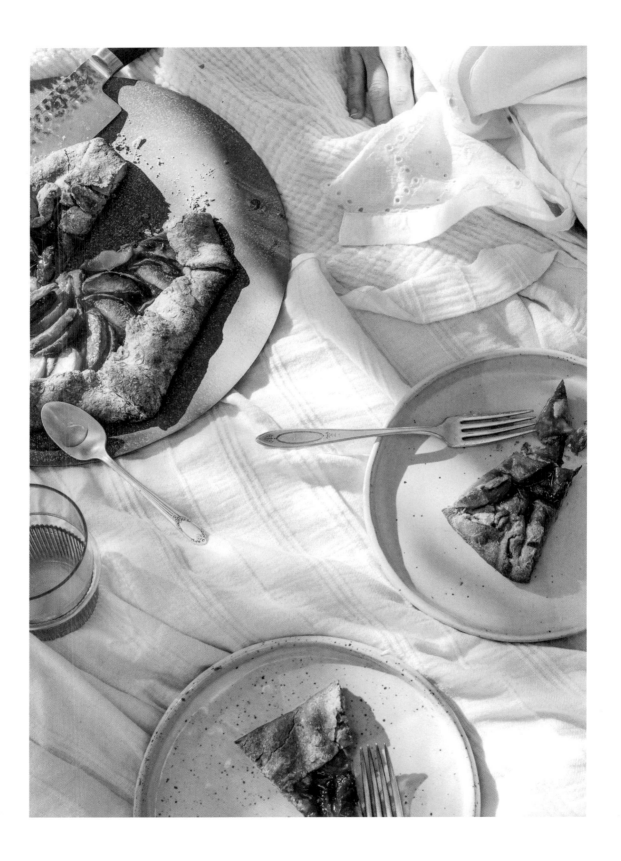

Rustic Fig Galette

I'll never forget the first fresh fig I tasted one summer—ripe and juicy right off the tree, warm from the afternoon sun. I wasn't just eating a piece of fruit; I was fully engaged in the sensory experience of bliss and delight in that moment. Fresh figs are one of those rare seasonal gifts I look forward to each year. If you can keep them around long enough to cook, this fig galette makes a perfect summer treat for a late afternoon picnic. Cooking figs into a jam makes them more digestible when paired with a grain, such as this galette crust. If figs aren't available in your area, this recipe format can be applied to any kind of seasonal summer fruit. My favorite variations include juicy peaches, blackberries, or raspberries.

PREP: 40 minutes | COOK: 30 minutes | YIELD: 6 servings

PASTRY DOUGH

2 cups oat flour or spelt flour

⅓ cup coconut sugar

¼ teaspoon salt

6 tablespoons cold ghee, cubed

3–4 tablespoons ice water

FILLING

10 fresh figs, stems removed

½ teaspoon ground cinnamon

½ lemon, juiced and zested

2 fresh figs, sliced into thin rounds for layering

Optional: Raw honey, for serving

Pulse the flour, coconut sugar, and salt in a food processor to combine. Add the cubed ghee slowly, and then the ice water. Process lightly until it begins to form a ball of dough. Remove from the food processor and shape dough into a round ball. Wrap in plastic and lightly press down on the dough to form a disk. Chill in the fridge for 20 minutes.

While the dough sets, prepare the filling. Combine the whole figs, cinnamon, lemon juice, and lemon zest in a small saucepan and cook on medium-low heat for 15 minutes, stirring regularly to avoid burning. Add a splash of water if needed. When the mixture has broken down into a jam, remove from heat and set aside.

Preheat the oven to 375°F. Remove the dough from the fridge and allow it to warm to room temp. Set a sheet of parchment paper on a flat surface and use a rolling pin to roll the dough out evenly onto the parchment sheet. Use extra flour on your rolling pin if you find the dough is sticking. Place the parchment with the rolled dough onto a baking sheet. Fill the center of the crust with the fig filling, leaving about 2 inches of dough around the edges. Arrange the sliced figs on top of the filling. Fold the edges of the dough onto the filling. Place in the oven and bake for 25–30 minutes, or until the crust is golden and slightly crispy. Remove from the oven and allow to cool. Drizzle a spoonful of raw honey on top before serving.

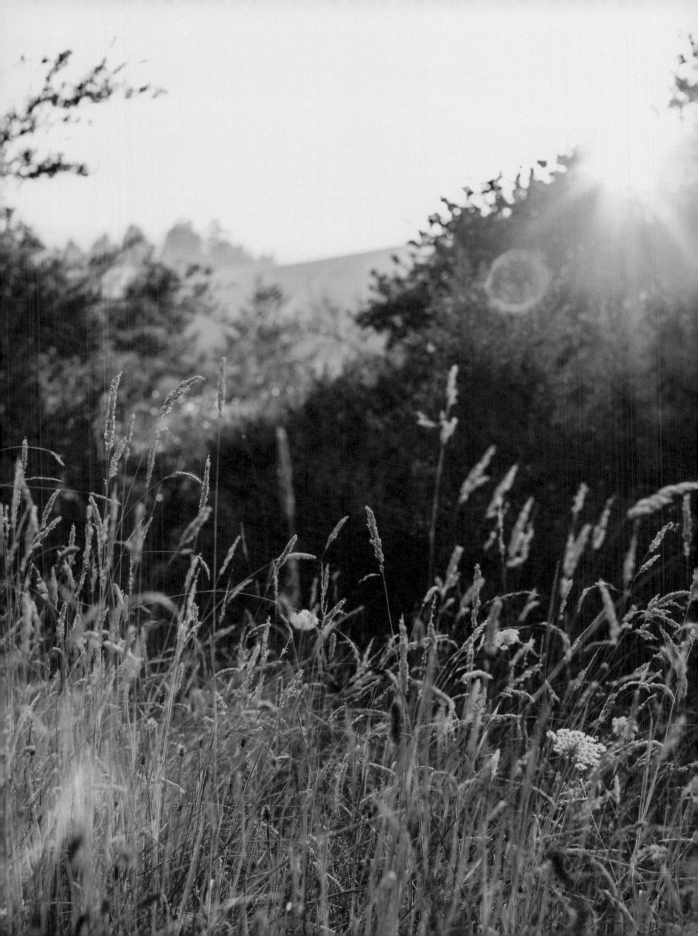

FALL

Fading light. Leaves turn. Let's head in and get cozy. Autumn is here.

Fall is vata season. The dry, rough, and mobile qualities must be balanced with stability, routine, and grounding. Accumulated heat and fatigue from summer's intensity can leave us feeling burnt out and more prone to anxiety. With the changing of the seasons, autumn is an especially important time to care for the nervous system and prioritize slowing down to support the transition from an active and outward summer toward a more restful, inward winter. A daily routine becomes more valuable than ever to support us in this seasonal transition. Your fall routine might include foods and practices that are warming, grounding, and stabilizing. Explore these restorative yoga practices, rituals for rejuvenation, and recipes that celebrate the abundance of fall's harvests with more soups, stews, and roasted vegetables.

Staying Balanced through Fall

EMPHASIZE

FOOD: Oily, soupy, warm, and well-cooked meals of whole grains, lentils, root vegetables, cooked greens, and stewed fruits; warming spices and healthy oils (ghee, untoasted sesame oil, mustard oil); stick to a consistent meal routine eaten with minimal distractions.

BREATH: Grounding and calming breathing that soothes anxiety and supports the nervous system, such as Nadi Shodhana or Sama Vritti pranayama that focuses on even, rhythmic inhalations and exhalations; try a steady ujjayi breath during asana.

MOVEMENT: Warming, stabilizing, and engaging movement with directed focus, shorter holds with some repetition; standing poses emphasizing grounding and balance, hip openers, gentle inversions, and long Savasana practiced in a warm, cozy environment.

MEDITATION: Mantra repetition to focus the mind, candle gazing, or a restorative yoga nidra meditation.

MINIMIZE

FOOD: Raw vegetables; bitter and astringent foods; cold smoothies and iced drinks; dried fruits and nuts; crackers, chips, and other dry snacking foods; caffeine or other nervous system stimulants; long periods of fasting or erratic eating.

BREATH: Cooling breathing, such as Sitali, or fast, sharp breathing that agitates the mind and nervous system.

MOVEMENT: Fast and mobile activities, cold or wind exposure, loud music or hyper-stimulating environments; exercise beyond 50–70 percent of your capacity.

Tips for Tending Your Inner Fire in Fall

With the transition from a hot summer to a cooler fall, your digestion may feel erratic or variable. Try these tips for balancing your inner fire:

- Skip all cold liquids and sip hot water between meals. Prepare a thermos of herbal tea to enjoy throughout the day. CCF Tea (page 65) works wonders if you feel bloated.

- Avoid grazing, skipping meals, or eating at irregular hours in the day. Prioritize a meal routine to stick to and eat without distraction.

- Always opt for cooked foods over raw. When your digestive fire is weak, keep to a simple diet of Kitchari (page 70) or Savory Breakfast Kanji (page 222) until you regain your hunger.

- Enjoy a warm spiced milk drink before bed, such as the Shatavari Rose Latte (page 216).

Fall Asana: *Grounding*

In this vata-balancing sequence, let your awareness move downward to the earth. With a series of standing postures that build strength in your legs and feet, calming forward folds, and inversions that draw energy out of your head, you'll leave this practice feeling more grounded and at ease. Calm your thinking mind with a steady gaze and attention to your breath and body. Allow this time on the mat to become a safe space for reflection, grounding, and unwinding. As you move through this practice, ask yourself, "What does stability feel like in my body and mind? How can I support myself to comfortably slow down?"

FALL PRACTICE TIPS

- Practice at a slow, smooth, fluid, and steady pace.

- Hold each posture for a short amount of time but with multiple repetitions.

- Protect your joints by hugging muscle to bone and finding stability in your legs.

- Keep a fixed gaze on the horizon to maintain balance and focus.

- Feel a connection to the earth through your feet and seat.

- Emphasize longer inhalations.

- Prioritize rest with a long restorative Savasana.

DOSHA NOTES

Ⓟ Move at a moderate pace. Incorporate soothing exhales through your mouth to release built-up heat, anger, or agitation.

Ⓚ Challenge yourself with longer holds in standing postures. Move through the seated series with moderate pace and deeper ujjayi breathing. End with a shorter Savasana.

TADASANA (MOUNTAIN POSE)

Stand with your feet hip-distance apart and your arms by your sides, eyes at the horizon. Feel all four corners of your feet rooted into the earth. Inhale, lengthen your spine long and lift through the crown of your head. Exhale, reach your fingertips toward the earth and bring energy into your arms. Draw your hands to prayer position at your heart center.

MODIFICATIONS
- Squeeze a block between your upper inner thighs for more stability.

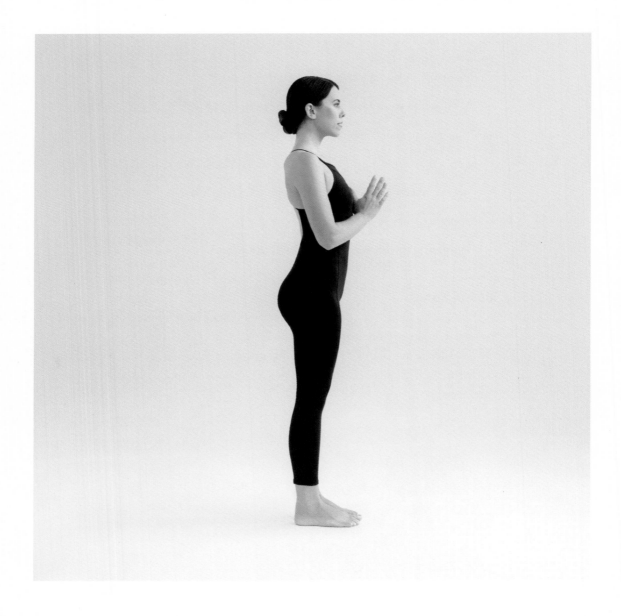

PARSVA URDHVA HASTASANA (SIDE BEND)

From Mountain Pose, reach your arms overhead and interlace your fingers with
your index fingers extended. Inhale, lengthen your spine. Exhale, slowly bend to the
right side. Press firmly into your feet and reach out through the crown of your head.
Inhale, return to center. Repeat on the left. Alternate bending side to side 2–3 times
in a fluid movement with the breath.

MODIFICATIONS

- Side bending can be as little or as deep as you comfortably move into.

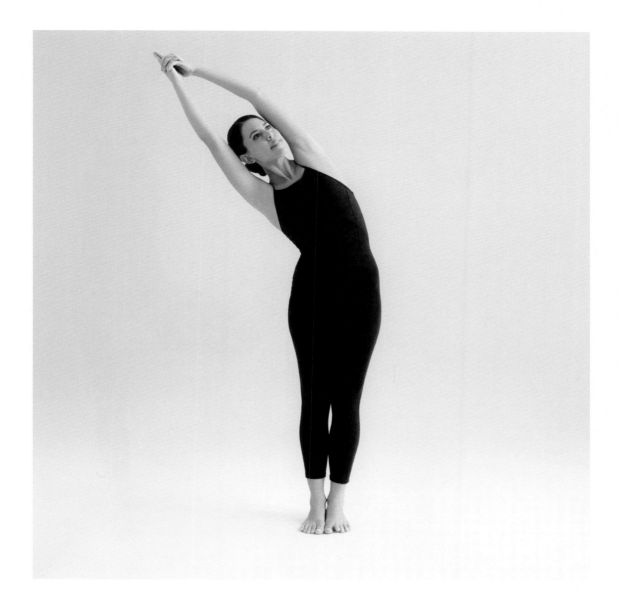

VRKSASANA (TREE POSE)

From Mountain Pose, lift your right knee to your chest. Rotate your knee out to the side and press your right foot to the inside of your left thigh, either above or below the knee joint, depending on your mobility. Press your palms together at your heart center and feel a lift in your chest, then extend your arms overhead. Balance and hold for a breath, then lower leg. Repeat on the left. Alternate balancing on both sides 2–3 times in a fluid movement with the breath.

MODIFICATIONS

- Use a wall or a chair to support balance.

- Place your foot on the ankle of your standing leg, with your toes on the floor to keep balance.

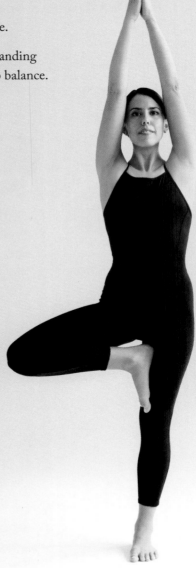

UTTANASANA (STANDING FORWARD BEND)

From Mountain Pose, inhale to lengthen your spine. Exhale, bend your knees slightly, and fold forward at your hips to lower your upper body toward your thighs. Release your hands toward the ground. Engage your quadriceps and lift your tailbone toward the sky. Release your head, neck, and shoulders toward the ground. Hold for 5–10 breaths.

MODIFICATIONS

- Bend your knees deeply to release tension from tight hamstrings.

- Rest your hands on a chair or two blocks six inches in front of your feet.

- Skip this posture if you have sciatic pain.

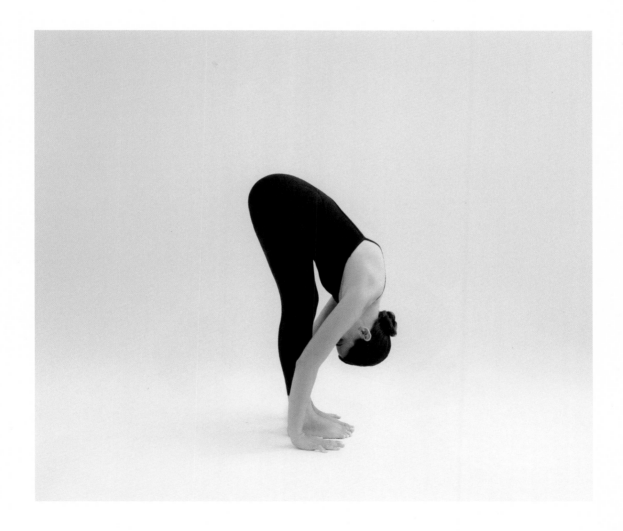

BALASANA (CHILD'S POSE)

Sit your hips back to your heels and lay your chest on your thighs. Place your forehead on the floor and draw your arms back by your feet, with palms facing up. Hold for 10 deep, slow breaths, or up to 5 minutes.

MODIFICATIONS

- Widen your knees and rest your chest between your legs. Extend your arms forward.

- Place a cushion or folded blanket between your calves and thighs for knee support.

- Rest your chest on a bolster for an even more restorative variation.

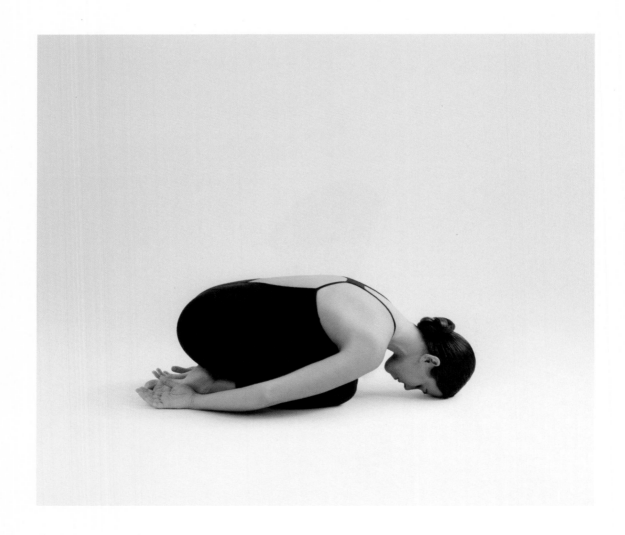

DANDASANA (STAFF POSE)

Sit upright with your legs extended straight in front of you. Inhale, lift your chest, lengthen your spine, and place your palms flat on the ground by your hips with your fingers pointing forward. Exhale, lengthen the back of your neck and draw your chin toward your chest. Hold for 5 breaths. Release and repeat 1–2 more times.

MODIFICATIONS

- Elevate your hips with a folded blanket.

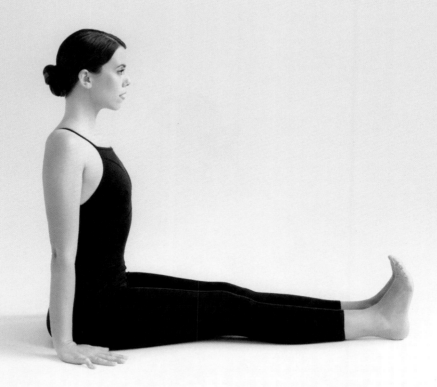

PASCHIMOTTANASANA (SEATED FORWARD FOLD POSE)

Sit upright with your legs extended straight in front of you. Flex your feet, pressing into the heels and balls of your feet to lengthen your legs. Inhale, and sit tall. Exhale, hinge at your hips to fold over your legs, and hold your ankles or wrap your hands around your feet. Hold for 5 breaths. Release and repeat 1–2 more times.

MODIFICATIONS

- Elevate your hips with a folded blanket. Use a strap or belt around your feet.

- Place a bolster or stack of pillows beneath your chest for a more restorative variation.

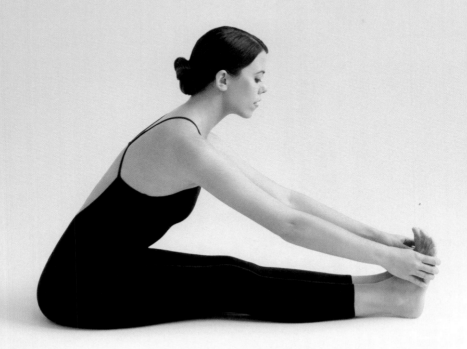

BADDHA KONASANA (BOUND ANGLE POSE)

Sit upright with your legs extended straight in front of you. Bend both knees and draw them toward your chest. Inhale, sit tall, and lengthen your spine. Exhale, open your knees to either side, and fold forward over your bent legs. Extend your chest over your feet. Hold for 5 breaths. Release and repeat 1–2 more times.

MODIFICATIONS

- Place pillows or blocks underneath each knee for support.

- Sit on a folded blanket or cushion to elevate your hips.

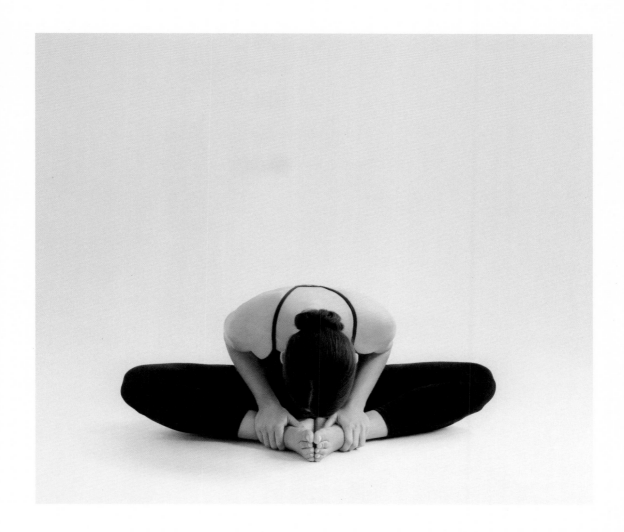

VIPARITA KARANI (LEGS AGAINST THE WALL)

Place a folded blanket, pillow, or bolster at a wall. Sit down with your hip at the wall to get your body as close as possible then lie down on your back. Extend your legs up the wall. Lift your hips and slide the support under your pelvis and low back, elevating your hips above your heart. Hold for 5–10 minutes.

MODIFICATIONS

- Place a small pillow or folded blanket under your neck for additional support.

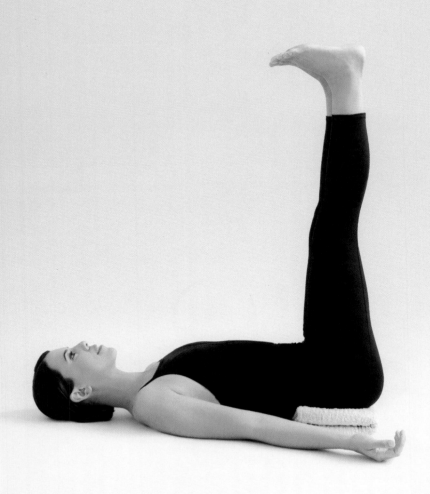

HALASANA (PLOW POSE)

Lie flat on your back, draw your knees into your chest. Press your palms into the floor and lift your hips over your shoulders. Bend your elbows and support your mid back with your hands. Draw your legs overhead, keeping your knees bent. Adjust your shoulders so you're resting on the top edges of your shoulders. Lengthen through the crown of your head to draw your chin away from your chest. Straighten your legs and press the balls of your feet into the floor. Hold for 5–10 breaths. When complete, release your arms by your sides, using them as support to roll down onto your back. Draw your knees to your chest and rest here for a few breaths.

MODIFICATIONS

- Use 1–2 folded blankets under your upper back and shoulders to take weight off your neck.

- Skip this posture if you have high blood pressure or glaucoma, or if you are pregnant or menstruating. Stay in Viparita Karani (Legs Against the Wall) for a gentler variation.

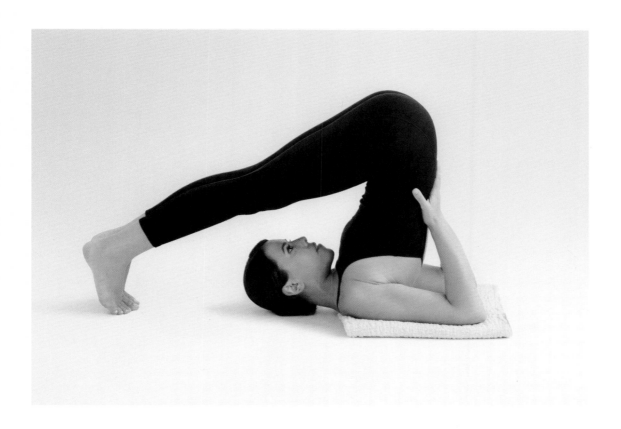

APANASANA (KNEES-TO-CHEST POSE)

Lie flat on your back and draw your knees into your chest. Wrap your hands around each knee or your forearms around your shins, grabbing hold of opposite wrists. Hold for 5–10 breaths.

MODIFICATIONS
- Place a folded blanket beneath your low back.

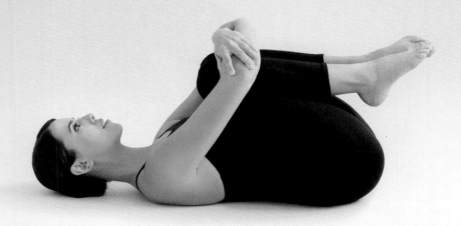

SAVASANA (CORPSE POSE)

The queen of all poses—do not skip this one! Set a gentle alarm if you're worried you may fall asleep. Lie on your back with your legs extended long and your arms resting by your side, palms up. Cover yourself with a blanket and support your joints by placing a pillow or bolster behind your knees. Cover your eyes with an eye pillow or cloth. Close your eyes, exhale deeply, and relax every inch of your body. Release any controlled effort to breathe. Rest in stillness for 10–15 minutes to complete your practice.

MODIFICATIONS
- Place an extra folded blanket or sandbag on your pelvis for weight, to soothe and ground your body.

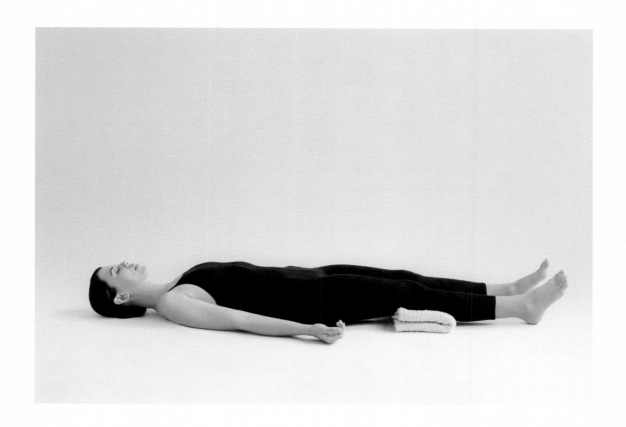

Fall Pranayama: *Nadi Shodhana*

Nadi Shodhana, or alternate nostril breathing, is the practice of clearing and harmonizing the subtle energy channels of the body. When you're feeling scattered, ungrounded, or overwhelmed, this gentle breathing practice works to balance the right and left hemispheres of your brain, soothe an overstimulated nervous system, and calm anxiety. This is an essential breath practice that benefits all three doshas, but it's particularly nourishing for vata dosha, especially in autumn. Try this as a way to start your day. Notice how it leaves you with more mental clarity and grounded energy.

HOW TO

On the physical level, you're breathing in and out of alternating nostrils. First, try a few rounds so you get the mechanics of this down. As you become more familiar with the movement of breathing through each nostril, then you can layer in a visualization. Imagine the breath (*prana*) moving from the ground up the right side of your spine as you inhale through your right nostril, and down the left side of your spine to the earth as you exhale through your left nostril. Repeat the visualization, ascending prana on each inhale and descending with each exhale.

1   Sit in a comfortable position that supports your spine and hips. This can be done cross-legged on the floor or upright in a chair. However you choose to sit, make sure your hips are relaxed and your head, neck, and spine are aligned. Relax your shoulders, neck, and jaw. Soften your belly.

2   Raise your right hand and extend your fingers. Cross your ring finger over your pinkie, fold your middle and index fingers down toward the palm and keep your thumb extended. This hand position forms *vishnu mudra*, the universal balance gesture. Keep your shoulders relaxed and your right elbow resting by your rib cage. Rest your left hand on your knee.

3   Take a deep breath through both nostrils. Using the thumb of your right hand, close your right nostril and empty the breath out of your left nostril.

4   Now close your left nostril with your ring finger. Inhale slowly through your right nostril. At the end of the inhale, close your right nostril with your thumb and exhale through the left. At the end of the exhale, pause for a moment and keep your left nostril open. Begin to inhale slowly through your left nostril, then close the left and open the right again to exhale. This completes 1 full round.

5   Repeat for 10 rounds total. You can also set a timer to practice this pranayama for 5 minutes, working up to 20 minutes a day.

6   When complete, bring both hands to rest on your knees and close your eyes. Take a few deep breaths through both nostrils and allow a few moments to quietly observe your body and mind before transitioning to movement.

PRACTICE NOTE

If you find it difficult to breathe through one nostril, try nasal irrigation with a neti pot (page 50) in the morning to relieve any congestion in the sinuses before practicing this pranayama. If you have a sinus infection, head cold, or acute nasal congestion, better to skip this pranayama and come back to it once your nose is clear.

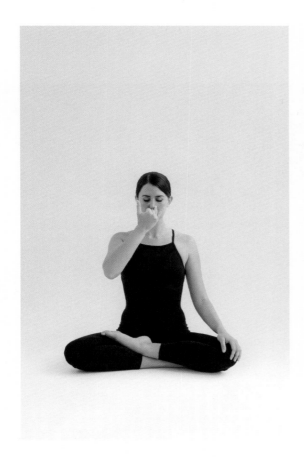
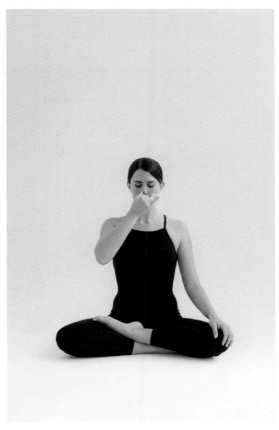

Fall Lunar Ritual: *Full Moon*

The full moon peaks vibrantly in the sky on the fourteenth or fifteenth day of the lunar cycle. The moon closest to the fall equinox is known as a harvest moon. This time of year, the moon will rise shortly after sunset, low on the horizon, giving it a radiant glow and magnificently large appearance. At the end of a long summer, the transition to fall welcomes the soothing, calming energy of the full moon. This ritual invites us to slow down while we make the very substance that helps feed our own vitality. Cooking is a creative act, and the full moon is often celebrated as a time to express our creativity.

WOMEN'S LUNAR RITUAL

The full moon is associated with ovulation, the peak of fullness and fertility. This is a playful time, a time for outward engagement and social activities. You might feel your most magnetic and charismatic. With pitta at its peak during ovulation, spend time in the full moon's rays and connect with your sensuality. Enjoy rich, sweet foods and herbs that boost fertility and support tissue rejuvenation—try the Ojas-Building Rice Drink (page 215), or Shatavari Rose Latte (page 216), or Warm Cinnamon Date Shake (page 219).

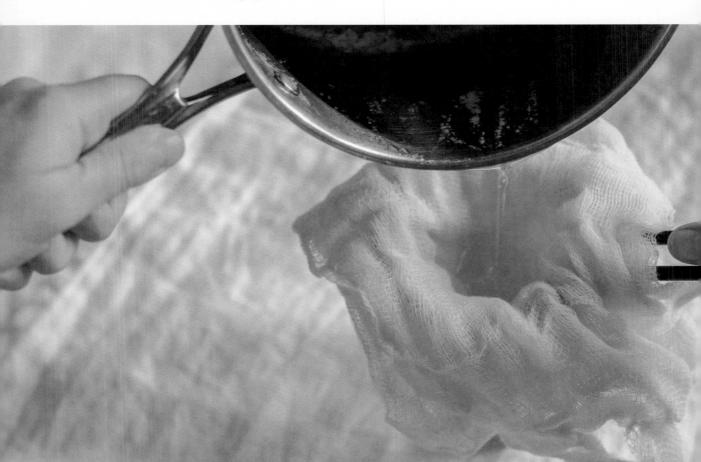

FULL MOON GHEE

Purnam in Sanskrit means "wholeness" or "fullness." *Purnima* is the day when the moon is full. Making ghee with the full moon is a beautiful monthly ritual to connect you with your own fullness and nourish you for the lunar cycle ahead. Chanting the Purnam Mantra while you slowly cook the ghee infuses this golden nectar with the vibration of the mantra. I like to make a large batch to stock my pantry for the month ahead.

WHAT YOU'LL NEED

2 pounds organic unsalted cultured butter

Heavy-bottomed stainless steel pot

Stainless steel spoon

Fine-mesh strainer

Clean glass jar

Optional: a tuning fork or singing bowl

THE RITUAL

Follow the instructions for making Ghee (page 66). The method is the same, yet the ritual invites you to take this beyond an ordinary kitchen day and into a place of meditation and devotion. You can simply prepare the ghee in silence, offer prayers or affirmations while you stir and skim, or consider chanting the mantra below. Once the ghee is made, place it on a windowsill to sit in the moonlight. Store it in a cool, dry place in your pantry or in the fridge. Use this special infused ghee for your cooking, from full moon to full moon.

> *OM Purnamadah Purnamidam*
> *Purnat Purnamudachyate*
> *Purnasya Purnamadaya*
> *Purnamevavashishyate*
> *OM Shanti Shanti Shanti*
>
> *That is the whole.*
> *This is the whole.*
> *From wholeness emerges wholeness.*
> *Wholeness coming from wholeness,*
> *Wholeness still remains.*
> *Peace in my heart, peace with each other, peace in the cosmos.*

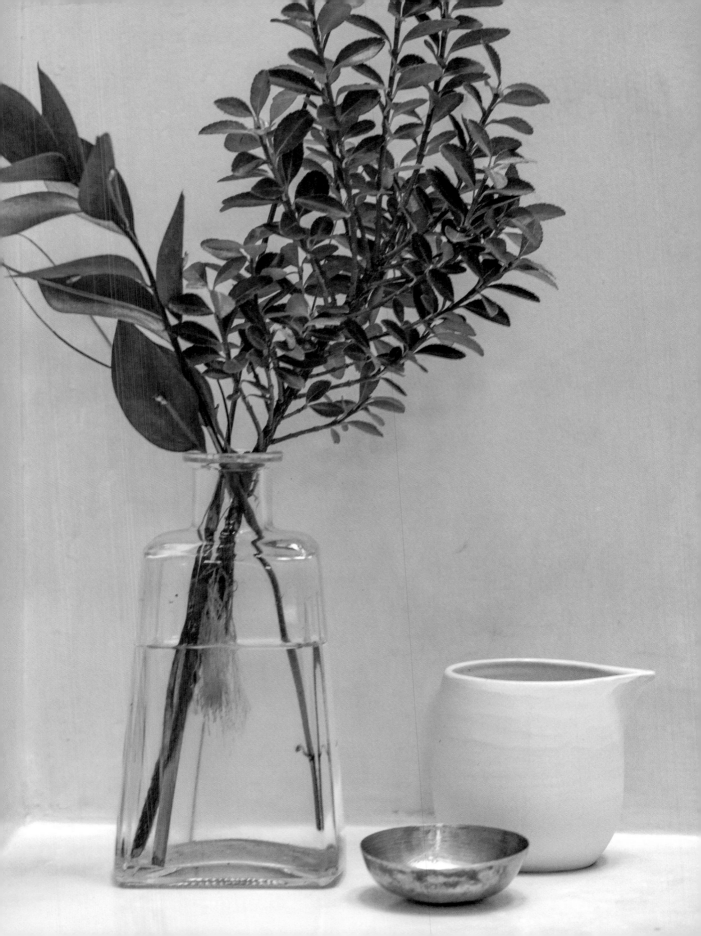

Fall Seasonal Ritual: *Equinox Cleanse*

After the sun peaks with the summer solstice, solar energy begins to wane and lunar energy increases with the fall equinox. This six-month cycle from the summer to winter solstice, known as *dakshinayana*, releases water and brings a much-needed cooling energy back to the earth. Autumn is marked by a sort of nostalgic change, a subtle entropy as all that peaked and bloomed returns to the earth in a quiet decay. In a similar way, we bloom and then turn back inward for a period of our own inner rejuvenation.

Cleansing at the fall equinox offers a time to release accumulated heat after a long summer and, most importantly, balance and nurture vata dosha. In a society that rarely slows down, this seasonal transition can bring feelings of anxiety and agitation. Popping and cracking in our joints, bloating, constipation, dry skin, and red eyes can be physical signs that it's time to support the body to come back into balance. Whereas the Spring Equinox Cleanse was all about deeper cleansing and releasing excess water, fall cleansing is about rejuvenating, building up your vitality, and boosting agni. *Rasayana*, which literally translates to "the pathway of vitality or juiciness," is the Ayurvedic term for rejuvenation practices. This ritual is about restoring juiciness through food, breath, movement, and nourishing self-care practices.

PREPARE

To prepare for this autumn rejuvenation, the most important thing to consider is timing. Look ahead to your calendar, between end-of-summer travels and winter holidays, and block off time where you can devote a weekend, a week, or even two weeks to rebalancing your routines. Limit your social engagements and travel commitments as much as possible in this sensitive seasonal transition; it will help you stay grounded and feel strong.

NOURISH

Your autumn diet shifts away from raw salads, cooling soups, and juicy fruit to hearty stews and oily cooked meals that are warm and well spiced. Incorporate more ghee and healthy fats into your diet. This seasonal ritual is less about losing weight, and more about ditching the habits that are detracting from your vitality. You know what I mean here—those little habits you picked up along the way to keep you going in busy times but that you know are now depleting you (think late nights and coffee-fueled days). Prioritize rest and slowing down. Try activities that are calming and soothing—think restorative yoga and walks in nature. This seasonal ritual is an opportunity to nurture yourself on a deep level.

YOUR DAILY CLEANSE ROUTINE

- Wake with the sun and set your intentions for the day.

- Instead of grabbing your phone, let your eyes gaze at something beautiful first—this could be fresh flowers, a yantra or pleasing piece of art, or something in nature—stay off all technology until you finish your morning practice and through the day, if possible.

- Follow your morning dinacharya practices (page 48).

- Drink a large glass of warm water with lemon.

- Prepare a pot of warming digestive tea to sip throughout the day.

- Try the Grounding Fall Yoga Sequence (page 191) and finish with 10 rounds of Nadi Shodhana pranayama (page 204).

- Eat at consistent times—breakfast by 8 a.m., lunch by noon, dinner by 6 p.m.—enjoy meals in silence.

- Wind down with a warm oil massage (page 51) and hot Epsom salt bath. Get in bed by 9 p.m. to wind down and be asleep by 10 p.m.

SAMPLE MENU

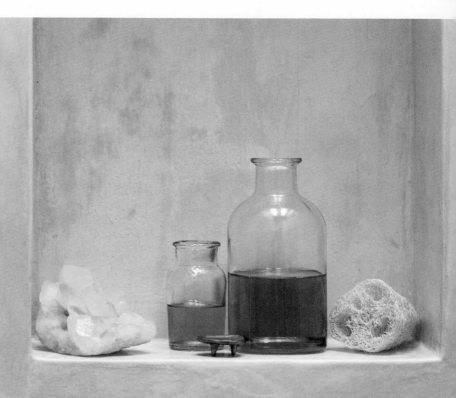

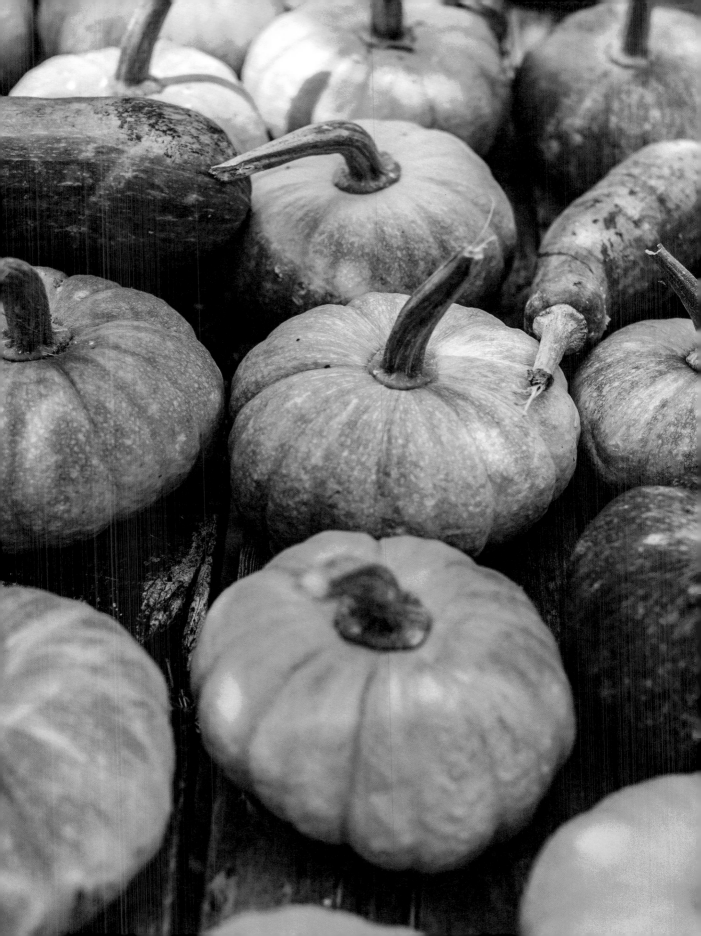

Fall Recipes

Shakti Chai

This chai gets the name Shakti because it's both potent and soft. It's laced with feminine herbs such as rose, shatavari, ashwagandha, and damiana. These herbs are wonderful reproductive tonics and rasayanas—rejuvenating substances. Try preblending the dry spices and storing in a jar out of direct sunlight to have a homemade chai mix ready for when cold mornings call for a warming drink.

PREP: 5 minutes | COOK: 30 minutes | YIELD: 4–6 servings

6–7 cups water

10 cardamom pods

2 cinnamon sticks

8 whole cloves

8 black peppercorns

1 tablespoon dried orange peel or the peel of 1 fresh orange

1 teaspoon cut shatavari root

½ teaspoon cut ashwagandha root

1 tablespoon dried damiana leaves

1 tablespoon dried rose petals

2 tablespoons fresh ginger, roughly chopped

Milk of your choice, ground cinnamon or nutmeg, and raw honey or maple syrup, for serving

In a medium pot, bring water to a boil on high heat. Using a mortar and pestle, crush the cardamom pods lightly to break them open and release their aromas, then crush the cinnamon sticks to break into smaller pieces. Add all ingredients to the pot, cover with a lid, reduce to medium-low heat, and simmer for 25–30 minutes. Strain the liquid and discard the pulp. Pour into a mug and serve hot with a splash of milk, a sprinkle of cinnamon or nutmeg, and a spoonful of honey or maple syrup to sweeten.

Note: Omit the shatavari, ashwagandha, and damiana from your blend if you are pregnant or breastfeeding. Always consult a doctor before incorporating new herbs or making diet changes if you are on medication.

Ojas-Building Rice Drink

For those with a vata constitution or vata imbalance, opting for snacks that provide warm and grounding nourishment can help reduce the dry, light, and rough qualities of vata dosha in fall. This warm rice drink makes a nourishing afternoon treat that's easy on the digestion. It's also a great way to use up any extra rice from a previous meal.

PREP: 5 minutes | COOK: 20 minutes | YIELD: 1–2 servings

1 cup cooked basmati rice

1–2 fresh Medjool dates, pitted

1 tablespoon ghee

¼ teaspoon ground cardamom

¼ teaspoon ground cinnamon

¼ teaspoon ground ginger

2 cups warm water

Combine all ingredients in a blender and puree until creamy. Enjoy warm or at room temperature.

DOSHA NOTES
Ⓟ Omit ginger.
Ⓚ Omit ghee.

Snacking the Ayurvedic Way

When we're in a pattern of habitual snacking, it's often because we haven't eaten enough at a meal, we skipped a meal altogether, or we're eating for entertainment and emotional comfort. In any of these events, eating when distracted can put the body in a stressed state and leave us with indigestion, bloating, and fluctuating energy levels. Of course, there are times when we may be more active, traveling, or simply needing more nourishment, and a snack is reasonable. In these times, it can be helpful to know which snacks will bring balance rather than depletion. Equally, building awareness and healthier routines around daily eating habits can take us out of the cycle of snacking as a lifestyle. In fall, selecting snacks that are warm, oily, well cooked, and hydrating is essential for nourishing vata dosha. Avoiding typical snack foods such as crackers, chips, popcorn, cookies, dried fruits, or excessive amounts of raw foods is a good rule of thumb.

Shatavari Rose Latte

Shatavari makes another appearance here in this late summer and fall recipe as a supportive rasayana, or rejuvenating substance, that can replenish your system and soothe pitta's effects. Known as "the queen of herbs," shatavari's bitter and sweet tastes cool down an overheated and depleted body after a long summer. It's also a wonderful reproductive tonic for both women and men through all stages of life.

PREP: 5 minutes | COOK: 5 minutes | YIELD: 1–2 servings

2 cups organic raw dairy milk or unsweetened rice or oat milk

1 teaspoon rose water

½ teaspoon shatavari powder

¼ teaspoon ground cardamom, plus more for garnish

1–2 teaspoons maple syrup

Optional: ½ teaspoon dried rose petals, for garnish

In a small saucepan, heat the milk to medium heat just to a boil. Transfer to a high-speed blender and add the rose water, shatavari, cardamom, and maple syrup. Blend until frothy. Pour into a mug and garnish with cardamom and dried rose petals, if using. Sip hot.

DOSHA NOTES

(K) Use almond milk.

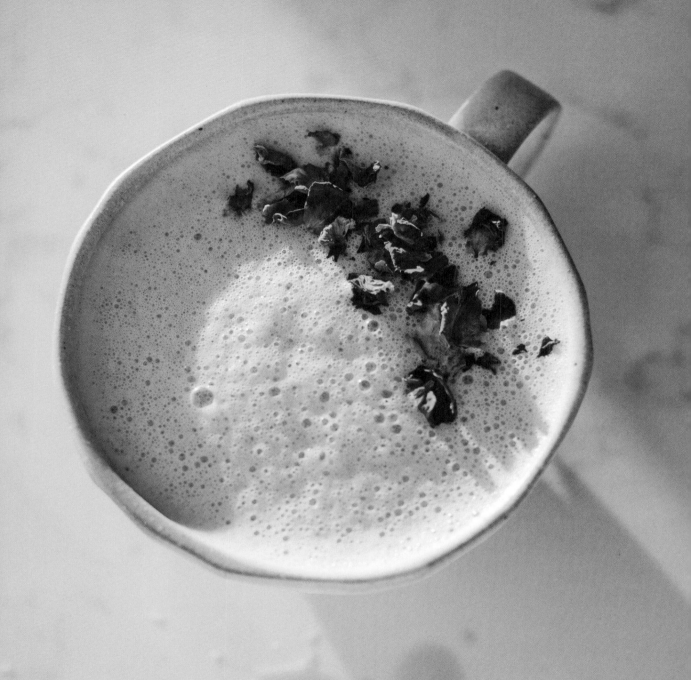

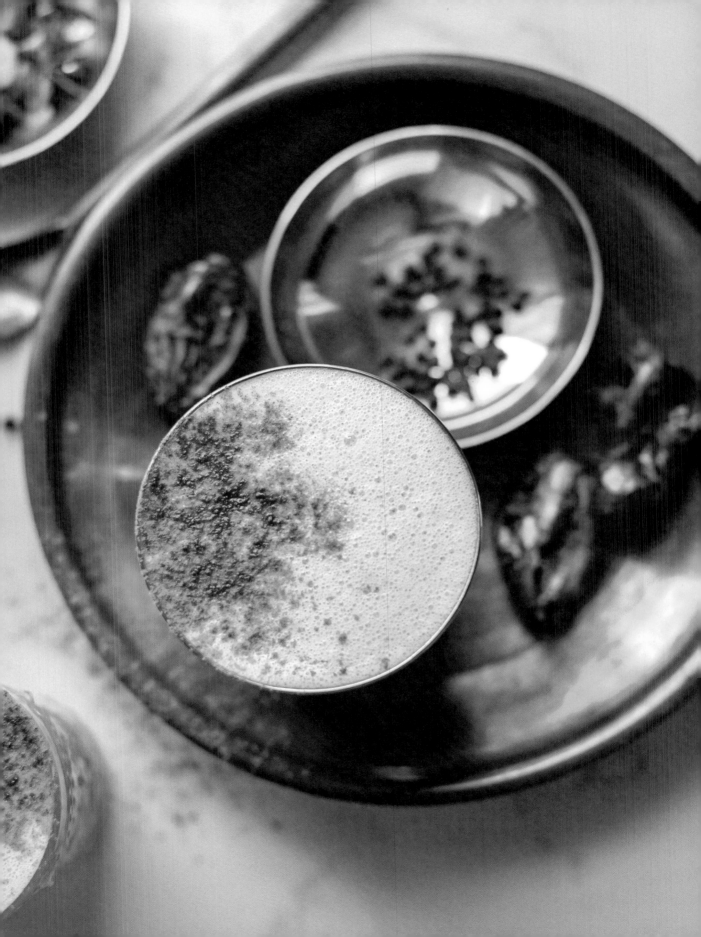

Warm Cinnamon Date Shake

This rich, warming date shake is a friend to cold-weather digestion. Where icy smoothies quickly dampen digestive fire, the combination of warming spices and sweet tastes nourish a depleted body and balance an anxious mind from excess vata in fall. Don't be put off by the cumin. It's surprisingly wonderful and subtle, pulling the whole drink together to balance the sweetness of the dates and milk.

PREP: 8–12 hours for soaking almonds | COOK: 5 minutes | YIELD: 1–2 servings

1 cup warm organic raw dairy milk or unsweetened rice or oat milk

10 raw almonds, soaked and peeled

1–2 Medjool dates, pitted

¼ teaspoon ground cinnamon

Pinch of ground cumin

Pinch of black pepper

In a small pot, heat the milk on low heat. Once hot, transfer to a blender. Combine remaining ingredients and blend until creamy. Pour into a glass and enjoy warm.

DOSHA NOTES

Ⓟ Omit black pepper.

Ⓚ Use almond milk.

Butternut Buckwheat Porridge

This porridge is a tried-and-true breakfast staple in my kitchen. It's my cold weather go-to from fall to late winter. There's something so grounding and satiating about a warm bowl of porridge, especially when cooked with sweet butternut squash or pumpkin and topped with warming cinnamon. On very dry and cold days I might add an extra spoonful of ghee to the mix for more vata support.

PREP: 5 minutes | COOK: 30 minutes | YIELD: 2–4 servings

3 cups water

½ cup buckwheat groats or short-grain brown rice

½ cup steel-cut oats

1 cup peeled butternut squash, cut into 1-inch cubes

¼ cup raisins

1 teaspoon ghee

1 teaspoon ground cinnamon

¼ teaspoon salt

Milk of choice and maple syrup, for serving

In a medium pot, combine all ingredients and bring to a boil on high heat. Cover with a lid, reduce heat to medium, and simmer for 30 minutes, until butternut squash is tender and grains are fully cooked. Toward the end, add a splash more water if needed. If using a pressure cooker, reduce the water to 2½ cups and follow instructions for pressure-cooking porridge. Once done, remove from heat and serve hot with a splash of milk of choice and a drizzle of maple syrup on top.

DOSHA NOTES

(P) Reduce cinnamon.

(K) Omit oats and double the buckwheat groats.

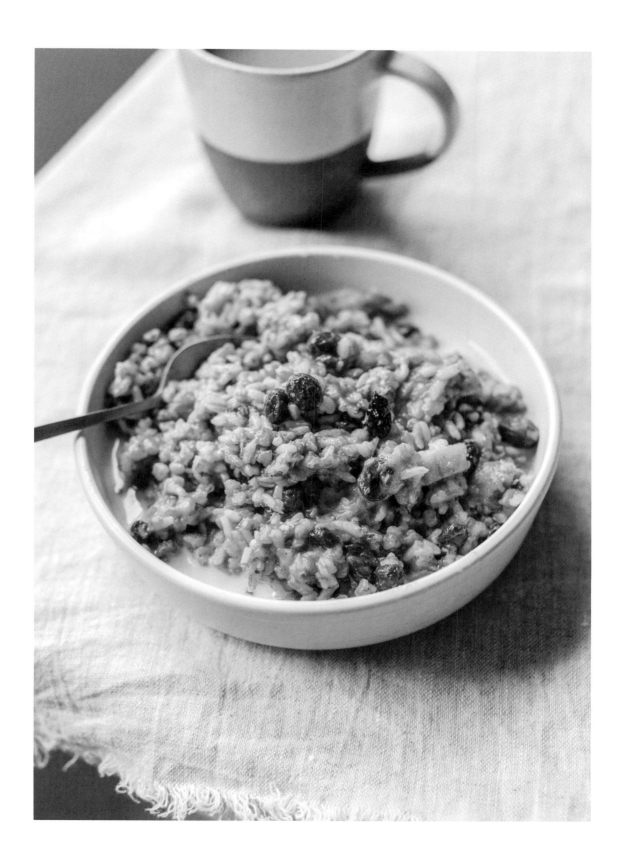

Savory Breakfast Kanji

Kanji, sometimes spelled *congee* in other Eastern cultures, is a watery rice porridge. It's often used as a healing dish in cleanse protocols, when recovering from illness, menstruating, or in the first weeks postpartum. But just as a bowl of oatmeal can be as simple or exciting as you'd like it to be, so too can kanji be an inviting canvas to create a variety of flavorful meals from this ultrasimple dish. Try the base porridge on its own or spice it up with this savory variation. This soupy, warm rice porridge is a perfect dish for balancing vata and boosting digestion.

PREP: 5 minutes | COOK: 90 minutes | YIELD: 2 servings

PORRIDGE

½ cup white basmati rice

5–7 cups water, plus more for rinsing the rice

½ teaspoon salt

SAVORY TOPPINGS

1 tablespoon ghee

1 inch fresh ginger, minced

½ teaspoon ground coriander

1 cup tightly packed spinach

¼ cup cilantro, finely chopped and divided

1–2 tablespoons white miso paste

1 tablespoon lime juice

1 teaspoon ume plum vinegar

1 teaspoon black sesame seeds

Optional: poached or fried eggs or fresh cooked fish

Add the rice to a large bowl and cover with water. Use your hands to stir the rice and rinse well, rubbing the rice in the palms of your hands. This is an important step that should not be skipped. Rinsing the rice helps remove any residue from the grains. The water will be murky. Drain, rinse, and repeat the washing 1 to 2 more times, until water is clear.

In a large pot with a thick bottom, add 5 cups water, the rinsed rice and salt, cover partially with a lid, and bring to a boil on high heat. Reduce to medium heat, cover and cook for 1–1½ hours, stirring occasionally to prevent sticking. This also makes it creamier. If you'd like a more watery porridge, add another 2 cups water and continue to cook until the desired consistency is reached. Remove from heat and keep warm until ready to serve.

In a skillet, melt the ghee. Stir in the ginger and coriander, and cook on medium heat for 1 minute, stirring frequently. Add the spinach and chopped cilantro (hold back some for garnish), stir to coat, and cook until slightly wilted, about a minute. Remove from heat and set aside. Add the miso paste, lime juice, and ume plum vinegar into the pot of cooked kanji and stir until well combined, then stir in the cooked spices and greens at the end. Garnish with cilantro and a sprinkle of black sesame seeds, to serve. For a heartier option, try this with a poached egg or a piece of fresh cooked fish.

DOSHA NOTES
Ⓟ Omit ume plum vinegar.
Ⓚ Omit ghee.

Immunity Broth

When I'm feeling run down or depleted, I make this deeply nourishing veggie broth to boost my immune system and rest my digestion. Alongside kitchari, this broth is a part of my autumn rejuvenation routine. Fast on the broth, use it as a stock in other recipes, or try blending the veggies into it for a creamy soup.

PREP: 10 minutes | COOK: 1 hour | YIELD: 4–6 servings

8–9 cups water

4 carrots, peeled and cut into 2-inch pieces

2 red potatoes, scrubbed and quartered

1 sweet potato, scrubbed and quartered

1 large beet, scrubbed, peeled, and quartered

4 stalks celery, trimmed and cut into 2-inch pieces

½ head red cabbage, roughly chopped

10 shiitake mushrooms (fresh or dried)

1 bunch parsley

1 bunch cilantro

2 tablespoons olive oil

3 inches fresh turmeric, roughly chopped

3 inches fresh ginger, roughly chopped

2 tablespoons lime or lemon juice

½ teaspoon salt

In a large pot, bring water to a boil. Add the vegetables, herbs, oil, and spices. Cover and simmer on medium heat for 30 minutes. Reduce heat to low and continue to cook for another 30 minutes, until vegetables are well broken down. Add more water if needed.

Remove from heat and season with lime or lemon juice and salt, tasting and adding more if desired. Strain the pulp from the liquid and sip the broth alone, or for a creamy soup, pour into a blender and puree. Serve hot.

DOSHA NOTES

Ⓟ Reduce or omit fresh ginger.

Ⓚ Omit oil.

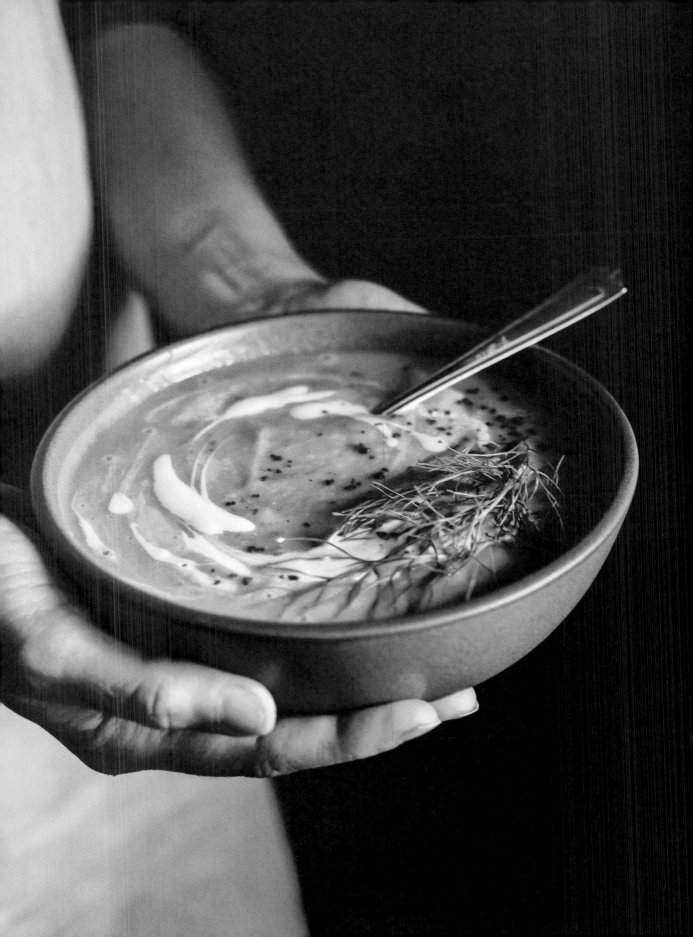

Kabocha Squash, Fennel & Red Lentil Soup

This rich soup incorporates the six tastes and yields a delicious, balanced Autumn meal. The fennel and fenugreek give it a maplelike sweet taste, while the red lentils provide protein and grounding nourishment with the squash. If you can't find kabocha squash, butternut or pumpkin work as wonderful alternatives.

PREP: 15 minutes | COOK: 40 minutes | YIELD: 4–6 servings

2 tablespoons ghee or olive oil

1 small fennel bulb, trimmed and sliced thinly; fronds reserved for garnish

1 tablespoon minced or grated fresh ginger

2 teaspoons ground turmeric

2 teaspoons ground coriander

1 teaspoon ground cumin

½ teaspoon ground fenugreek

3 cups cubed kabocha squash, peeled and deseeded

1 cup red lentils, rinsed well

1 teaspoon salt

5–6 cups water

1 tablespoon white miso paste

2 tablespoons lemon juice

Plain yogurt, for serving

In a medium pot, heat the ghee on medium-low heat. Add the fennel and sauté until tender. Add the ginger and cook another 1–2 minutes, until fragrant. Add the spices and stir to coat the fennel. Add the kabocha squash, stir to coat, and cook another 3–4 minutes. Last, add the red lentils, salt, and water. Cover and cook on medium heat for 40 minutes. Stir occasionally, adding more water if needed. Once the lentils and squash are tender, almost mushy, remove from heat and stir in the miso paste and lemon juice. Transfer to a blender and puree until creamy. Taste and adjust seasonings as needed. Serve hot with a swirl of yogurt and fennel fronds on top.

DOSHA NOTES
(P) Reduce ginger.
(K) Reduce oil.

Creamy Miso Tahini Dal

This Asian spin on a basic dal uses miso and tahini for a creamy soup. Serve with rice and greens for a nourishing meal. A note when shopping: remember to buy split yellow mung dal, not yellow split peas; they are two different beans with very different cook times.

PREP: 2 hours for soaking | COOK: 25 minutes | YIELD: 4 servings

4 cups water

1 cup split yellow mung dal, soaked 2 hours

1½ tablespoons white miso paste

1½ tablespoons tahini

½ lemon, juiced

Cooked brown or basmati rice, for serving

Chopped cilantro, for garnish

In a medium saucepan, bring water to boil, add the split yellow mung dal, and cook the dal on medium heat until soft, about 20 minutes. At the end, add the miso paste and tahini and stir until creamy. Add a little more water if needed. The consistency should be that of a creamy, thick soup. Serve over a scoop of brown or basmati rice, with chopped cilantro and a cooked veggie of your choice.

Delicata, Wild Rice & Pomegranate Salad

Pomegranates are a great end-of-summer and early fall fruit, helping to reduce pitta and circulate the blood and lymph. This antioxidant-rich wild rice salad makes a wonderful side dish to a holiday feast. When using delicata squash, you can leave the skins on for texture and extra nutrients.

PREP: 10 minutes | COOK: 50 minutes | YIELD: 4 servings

WILD RICE

1 cup wild rice

3 cups water

Pinch of salt

ROASTED SQUASH

1 small delicata squash, deseeded and cut into ¼-inch-thick half-moons

2 tablespoons olive oil

Pinch of salt

VINAIGRETTE

¼ cup olive oil

2 tablespoons apple cider vinegar

1½ teaspoons raw honey

1 teaspoon Dijon mustard

½ teaspoon ground turmeric

½ teaspoon salt

SALAD

1 cup pomegranate seeds

2 tablespoons thinly sliced scallions

½ cup chopped pistachios

¼ cup pumpkin seeds

1 cup microgreens

Optional: 2 ounces goat cheese

In a medium saucepan, combine the wild rice, salt, and water. Cover with a lid and bring to a boil over high heat, then reduce to medium-low and cook for 40–45 minutes. You will know the rice is done when some of the grains burst open. Drain excess liquid and set aside to cool.

For the squash: Preheat the oven to 400°F. Line a baking sheet with parchment paper and arrange the squash on the pan. Drizzle with olive oil and sprinkle with salt. Roast for 15 minutes, then flip squash over. Continue to roast for another 10–15 minutes, or until golden and tender. Remove from the oven and set aside to cool while you assemble the rest of the salad.

For the vinaigrette: Combine all ingredients in a jar, cover with a lid, and shake until well combined. Taste and adjust seasonings as needed. Set aside until ready to use.

In a large serving bowl, combine the wild rice, squash, pomegranate seeds, and scallions. Toss with half the dressing. Add the remaining seeds, nuts, and goat cheese, if using, and drizzle with remaining dressing. Serve immediately and enjoy warm.

DOSHA NOTES

Ⓟ Reduce apple cider vinegar.

Ⓚ Omit goat cheese.

Roasted Roots & Brussels Sprouts

Moving into fall and winter, you'll notice many of the salad recipes consist of more roasted vegetables than raw. This is intentional. Cooked food is more pacifying for vata and kapha, and generally easier to digest. This warming and grounding roasted roots and brussels sprouts works as a salad when served on top of a bed of greens or as a wonderful side dish that can be added to any autumn balanced bowl.

PREP: 15 minutes | COOK: 40 minutes | YIELD: 4 servings

ROOT VEGGIES

½ small kabocha squash, cut into 1-inch wedges with the skin on

2 small beets, scrubbed, trimmed, and quartered

2 medium turnips, scrubbed, trimmed, and quartered

12 brussels sprouts, trimmed and halved

2 tablespoons olive oil

Pinch of salt

Cracked black pepper

DRESSING

Small lime wedge

¼ cup olive oil

1 garlic clove

2 tablespoons lime juice, or to taste

1 teaspoon raw honey

2 tablespoons finely chopped cilantro

2 tablespoons finely chopped parsley

½ teaspoon salt

Cracked black pepper, to taste

Preheat oven to 425°F. Line a baking sheet with parchment paper and spread the veggies across the pan. Drizzle with olive oil and lightly toss to coat. Sprinkle with salt. Roast for 35–40 minutes, or until veggies are tender and golden on the edges. Remove from the oven, transfer to a large serving bowl and toss with dressing. Serve warm.

For the dressing: On a cutting board, squeeze the lime wedge. Hold the base of the fork with one hand and press it flat onto the board in the lime juice. With the other hand, grate the clove of garlic on the edges of fork prongs into a finely grated pulp. The acidity of the lime juice will cut the pungency of the garlic. Scoop up the grated garlic with a knife and place it into a bowl. Add the remaining ingredients and stir together. Once the roasted veggies are done, drizzle over top and serve hot.

DOSHA NOTES

Ⓟ Omit garlic; swap honey for maple syrup.

Ⓚ Enjoy with fresh arugula.

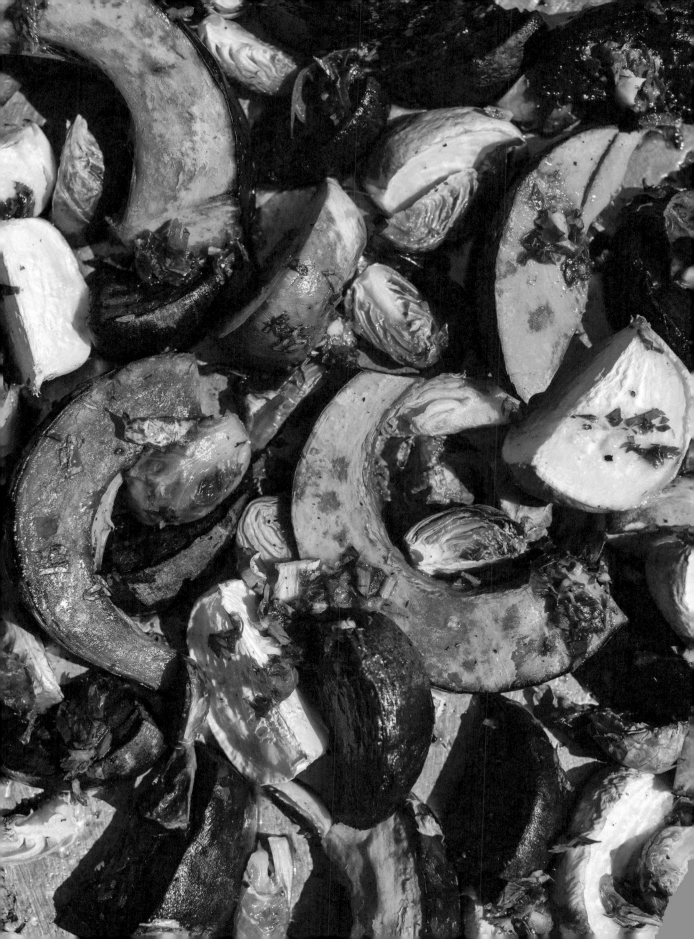

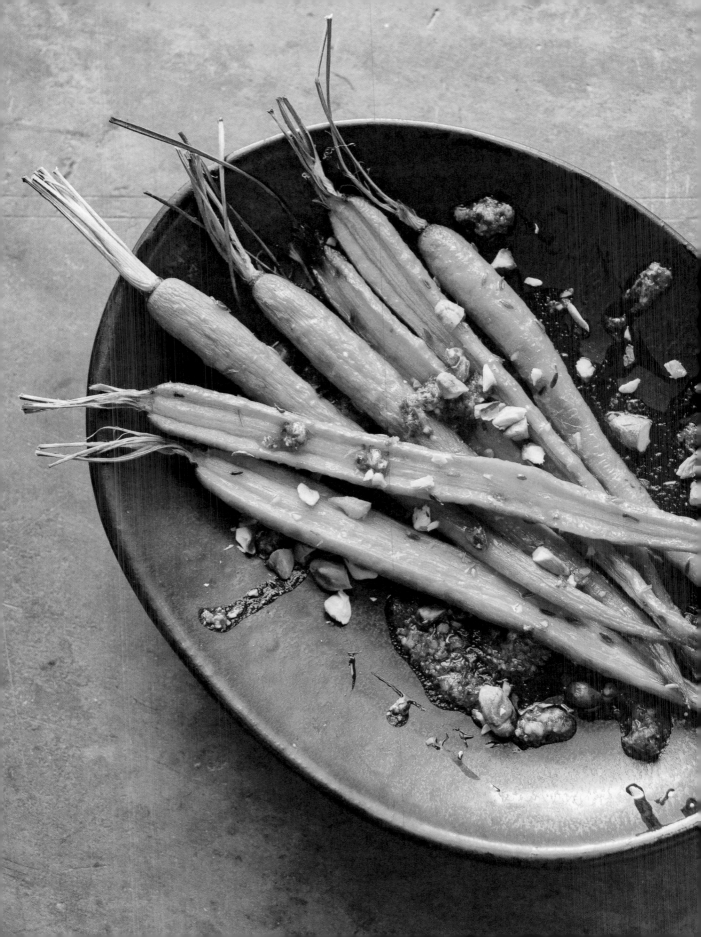

Cumin-Roasted Carrots with Carrot Top Gremolata

While this recipe can really be an all-season staple, I get excited in summer and early fall to find vibrant colorful carrots at the market with their long leafy greens intact. If you're buying them with their leafy tops, save these to add into a gremolata, pesto, or simple veggie broth. The fresh herb-and-bitter-greens gremolata make this dish a great addition for pitta and kapha. When roasted, carrots become sweet and grounding for vata.

PREP: 10 minutes | COOK: 25 minutes | YIELD: 4 servings

CUMIN-ROASTED CARROTS

6 whole carrots, green tops intact

1 tablespoon olive oil

1 teaspoon maple syrup

1 teaspoon cumin seeds

Pinch of salt

CARROT TOP GREMOLATA

1 cup roughly chopped carrot tops

½ cup roughly chopped parsley

½ cup mint

½ cup pumpkin seeds, or pistachios

¼ teaspoon salt

2 tablespoons lime juice

¼ teaspoon ground cumin

½ cup olive oil

Preheat the oven to 425°F. Scrub and rinse the carrots well. Remove the green tops and set aside for the gremolata. Slice carrots in half lengthwise. Spread across a parchment-lined baking sheet. Sprinkle with olive oil, maple syrup, cumin seeds, and salt. Roast in the oven for 20–25 minutes, or until tender and slightly crispy on the edges. Serve warm alongside your favorite balanced bowl or as a side dish with carrot top gremolata.

For the gremolata: Combine the carrot tops and herbs in a food processor. Pulse until broken down. Add the pumpkin seeds, salt, and lime juice. Blend again until well combined and smooth. Last, add the olive oil and pulse a few times to incorporate. Taste and adjust seasonings. Store in an airtight jar in the fridge for up to 3 days until ready to use.

Pumpkin Empanadas with Cashew Crema

These little empanadas are made from chapati dough and stuffed with savory fall flavors. Though a bit more labor intensive than a one-pot meal, this recipe makes for a fun addition to any holiday gathering or dinner party menu.

PREP: 1 hour | COOK: 30 minutes | YIELD: 12 servings

CHAPATI DOUGH (PAGE 73)

ROASTED PUMPKIN

4 cups cubed pumpkin or butternut squash (1-inch cubes)

1 tablespoon olive oil

Pinch of salt

Fresh cracked black pepper, to taste

FILLING

2 tablespoons ghee or olive oil

2 tablespoons minced shallot

2 cloves garlic, minced

8 shiitake mushrooms, stems removed and finely chopped (about ½ cup)

2 teaspoons curry powder

½ teaspoon ground cinnamon

⅛ teaspoon ground nutmeg

4 lacinato kale leaves, finely chopped (about ¾ cup)

2 tablespoons fresh thyme leaves, plus more for garnish

½ teaspoon salt

¼ teaspoon fresh cracked black pepper

To make the empanada dough, follow the instructions for Chapati. If your dough looks dry, add a little more water to the mixture as needed. Certain flours might yield different textures; this works best with whole wheat pastry flour. Place the dough in a bowl, cover with a towel, and allow to sit for 30 minutes at room temperature. When ready, roll out the dough on a floured surface. Use a 3-inch round cookie cutter or ring mold to stamp the dough into rounds. Take the scraps and press them into a ball, then roll out again into a flat sheet to stamp the remaining dough. Set aside the dough rounds until ready to assemble.

Preheat the oven to 350°F. Spread the cubed pumpkin across a baking sheet. Lightly coat in olive oil, and sprinkle with salt and pepper. Roast for 15–25 minutes, until tender; check after 10 minutes and toss. Note: butternut squash will cook quicker than pumpkin. Transfer to a bowl and mash with a fork. Set aside. Keep the oven on.

While the pumpkin is roasting, prepare the rest of the filling. In a medium skillet, heat the ghee over low heat, add the shallot and garlic, and sauté for 1–2 minutes until golden. Add the mushrooms, curry powder, cinnamon, and nutmeg. Cook for 5 minutes on low heat. Add the kale and cook another 2–3 minutes, until tender. Remove from heat and set aside. Mix the sautéed mushrooms, thyme, and salt and cracked black pepper to taste into the squash until fully incorporated. You want the consistency mostly smooth with some texture. Set the filling aside until ready to assemble.

CASHEW CREMA

1 cup cashews, soaked 1 hour

¾ cup water

1½ tablespoons apple cider vinegar

1 teaspoon fresh thyme leaves

1 clove garlic

1–2 tablespoons lime juice

1 teaspoon maple syrup

½ teaspoon salt

Pinch of ground nutmeg

For the cashew crema: Combine all ingredients in a high-speed blender. Puree until creamy. Taste and adjust seasonings as needed. Store in an airtight jar in the fridge for up to 3 days until ready to use.

To assemble, spoon about 1 tablespoon of filling into the center of each dough round. Fold one half over the other, lining up the edges. Use a fork to press down around the edges to seal the dough pocket. Arrange the empanadas on a baking sheet. Brush the tops with melted ghee or olive oil. Place in the oven and bake for 14–18 minutes at 350°F until golden brown. Serve warm right out of the oven with a drizzle of cashew crema and a sprinkle of fresh thyme.

DOSHA NOTES

(P) Use sunflower seeds in place of cashews for crema; omit garlic.

(K) Enjoy the dipping sauce in moderation.

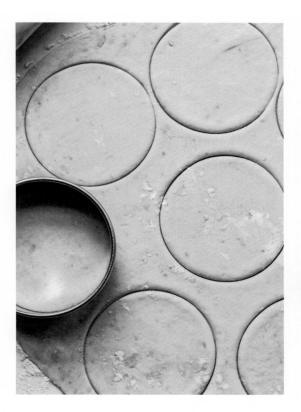
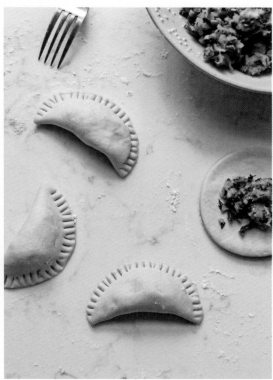

Autumn Quinoa Bowl with Turmeric Tahini Sauce

My roommates in college were from Beirut, so we spent many evenings together eating incredible home-cooked Lebanese food. They had a big influence on my culinary tastes, and you'll now find my pantry always stocked with za'atar, sumac, saffron, and fresh tahini. This autumn quinoa bowl combines my favorite Lebanese flavors with a creamy tahini sauce on top, all nourishing ingredients for grounding in autumn. Don't be intimidated by the longer recipe format. While there are several components to this bowl, the preparation itself is quite easy and is actually designed to be deconstructed and used in a variety of different ways.

PREP: 25 minutes | COOK: 30 minutes | YIELD: 4 servings

LEMON-ROASTED CAULIFLOWER

½ head of cauliflower, cut into small florets

1 tablespoon olive oil

2 tablespoons fresh lemon juice

Salt and fresh cracked black pepper

TOASTED CHICKPEAS

2 cups chickpeas, drained and rinsed

1 tablespoon extra-virgin olive oil

1 tablespoon ground sumac

½ teaspoon ground cumin

½ teaspoon sea salt, or to taste

Freshly ground black pepper

Preheat the oven to 400°F. Toss the cauliflower in olive oil and arrange in a single layer on half of a baking sheet. Drizzle with lemon juice and sprinkle with salt and pepper. Roast 25–30 minutes, until lightly golden and crispy. Keep warm until ready to serve.

While the cauliflower is roasting, prepare the chickpeas. Line a rimmed baking sheet with parchment paper. Spread the chickpeas out on a towel and pat dry until the towel has absorbed all the moisture from the chickpeas. In a large bowl, whisk together the olive oil, spices, and salt and pepper to taste. Add the chickpeas and toss well to coat. Transfer the seasoned chickpeas to the baking sheet and arrange in a single layer. Roast for 15–20 minutes, checking halfway through to shake and turn the pan. Remove from the oven once the chickpeas are golden and crispy.

SAFFRON QUINOA

2½ cups water

1 cup dry quinoa

4–6 threads saffron

1 tablespoon olive oil

2 tablespoons lemon zest

¼ teaspoon salt

TURMERIC TAHINI SAUCE

¼ cup tahini

2 tablespoons white miso paste

½ inch fresh ginger

1 tablespoon tamari

½ teaspoon ground turmeric

2 tablespoons fresh lemon juice

¼–½ cup water

Microgreens and chopped
cilantro, for garnish

For the quinoa: In a medium pot, bring water to a boil. Add the dry quinoa, saffron, and olive oil and simmer on medium heat until water is fully absorbed and quinoa is tender, about 20 minutes. Stir in the lemon zest. Season with salt.

For the sauce: Combine all ingredients in a high-speed blender and blend until creamy. Pour into an airtight container to store until ready to use. Stores up to 7 days in your fridge.

To serve, layer each bowl the warm quinoa, roasted cauliflower, and toasted chickpeas in a bowl. Drizzle the sauce over top and garnish with a handful of microgreens and cilantro.

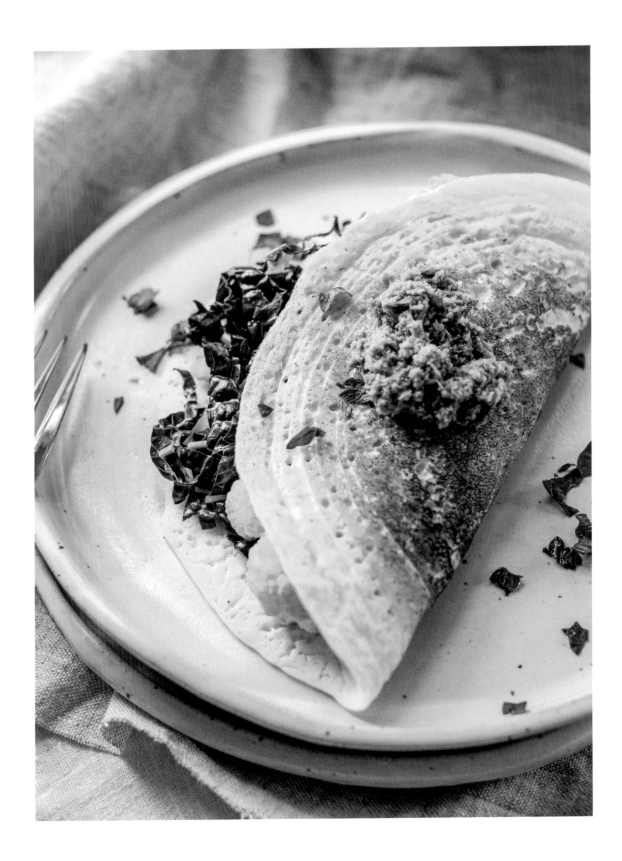

Aloo Gobi Masala Dosa

In Mysore, masala dosas are savory crepes stuffed with a spicy potato mixture. This fall version combines fennel and cauliflower to bring a sweetness to the dish that balances pitta and vata. Dosas are versatile, so try this with different veggies or chutneys to mix it up. Skip the fork and knife: my favorite way to enjoy dosas are with my hands.

PREP: 2 days for making dosa batter | COOK: 1 hour | YIELD: 4–6 servings

DOSAS (PAGE 72)

ALOO GOBI FILLING

1 small head cauliflower, trimmed and torn into small florets

2 red potatoes, cubed

1 fennel bulb, trimmed and sliced thinly

4 tablespoons olive oil

2 tablespoons curry powder

½ teaspoon ground fenugreek

½ teaspoon salt

1 tbsp fresh lemon juice

5–6 kale leaves, stems removed and chopped

COCONUT CILANTRO CHUTNEY

1 bunch cilantro, stems included

2–3 tablespoons lemon juice

½ cup water

1 cup unsweetened shredded coconut

1 inch fresh ginger

2 teaspoons raw honey

½ teaspoon salt

Follow the instructions for making Dosa. Once the batter is ready, cook the dosas while the veggies are roasting.

For the filling: Preheat the oven to 400°F. Combine all the vegetables in a large baking pan and toss with olive oil, spices, and salt. Roast for 35–40 minutes, or until tender and slightly crispy. Remove from oven.

Heat a skillet with 1 teaspoon ghee or olive oil, add the chopped kale and sauté until tender. Remove from heat and fold into the roasted veggie mixture. Serve hot.

For the chutney: While the veggies are roasting, prepare the chutney. Add cilantro, lemon juice, and water to a high-speed blender. Pulse until broken down. Add the remaining ingredients and blend into a paste. If the mixture is dry, add more water. Taste and adjust seasonings as desired. Transfer to a jar and store in the fridge for up to 3 days.

To assemble, plate the vegetables and chutney on the side, serve with a platter of hot dosas on the table. You can also fill the individual dosa with the vegetables and top with chutney.

DOSHA NOTES
- (P) Reduce curry powder.
- (K) Try turnips instead of potatoes.

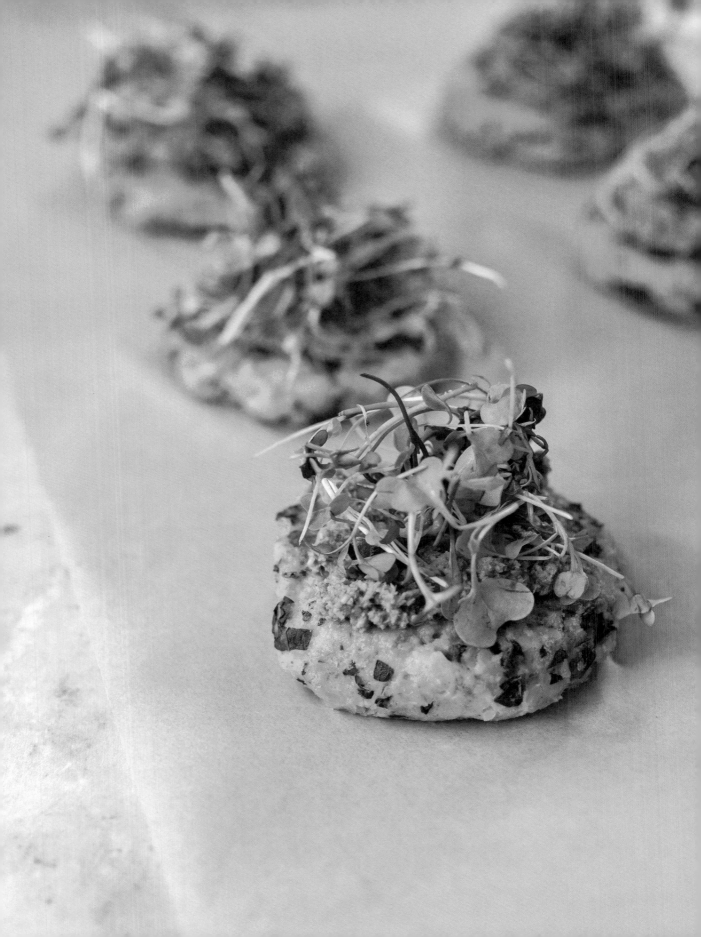

Kitchari Burgers

Switch up your basic kitchari and turn it into a burger! Instead of using leftover kitchari, try this deconstructed version using sushi rice instead of basmati. Sushi rice has a stickier texture than basmati, making it a great binder in place of the egg you often see in veggie burger recipes. I serve this with avocado and a spoonful of Coconut Cilantro Chutney.

PREP: 20 minutes | COOK: 45 minutes | YIELD: Makes 8 servings

KITCHARI BASE

½ cup split mung dal

½ cup sushi rice

¼ teaspoon salt

1 tablespoon ghee or sunflower oil

2½ cups water

BURGER MIXTURE

2 tablespoons ghee or sunflower oil, divided

1 tablespoon minced fresh ginger

2 tablespoons cumin seeds

1 tablespoon ground coriander

1 tablespoon ground turmeric

4 kale leaves, stems removed and finely chopped

1 cup cubed sweet potato, boiled and mashed

¼ cup cilantro, finely chopped

2 tablespoons ground flax

½ teaspoon salt

1 tablespoon lime or lemon juice

Optional: avocado slices, sprouts, and Coconut-Cilantro Chutney (page 237) for serving

For the kitchari: In a small pot, combine the mung dal, rice, salt, ghee, and water. Bring to a boil and cook on medium-high heat for 20–25 minutes, until water is fully absorbed and the mixture is thick and sticky. Transfer to a large mixing bowl and allow to cool.

For the burger: In a large skillet, heat the ghee and ginger on low heat. Add the remaining spices and kale. Sauté until cooked down, about 1–2 minutes. Transfer to a mixing bowl and fold the cooked spices and greens into the cooled kitchari base. Add in the mashed sweet potato, cilantro, flax, and salt. Drizzle the lime juice over top. Mix until well combined. Using wet hands, form a 3-inch ball into your hands and then light press into a patty. Repeat until you've formed 8 patties.

Heat a skillet on medium-high with a little bit of ghee or sunflower oil to grease the pan. Place the patties on the hot surface and cook until crispy and golden on one side, about 2–3 minutes. Flip and cook for another 3–5 minutes, until cooked through and golden on both sides. You may need to work in batches, depending on the size of your skillet. Serve warm with a slice of avocado, a handful of sprouts, and spoonful of Coconut-Cilantro Chutney.

Fall Harvest Muffins with Whipped Cinnamon Butter

This recipe made its way into my world first as a cake, then over the years evolved into my favorite hearty breakfast muffins. They are dense and packed with vata-balancing spices. Serve them in the morning or as an afternoon treat alongside a piping hot mug of chai.

PREP: 20 minutes | COOK: 25 minutes | YIELD: 12 servings

DRY INGREDIENTS

3 cups oat flour

1 cup coconut sugar

1 teaspoon baking soda

1 tablespoon ground cinnamon

½ teaspoon ground nutmeg

¼ teaspoon ground ginger

¼ teaspoon salt

WET INGREDIENTS

3 cage-free organic eggs,
or ½ cup flax whisked into
1 cup water

½ cup melted ghee or olive oil

1 tablespoon vanilla

1 cup grated zucchini

1 cup grated carrot

1 cup grated apple

6 dates, pitted and chopped

¼ cup walnut pieces

**WHIPPED CINNAMON
BUTTER**

4 ounces softened organic
cultured butter

1 tablespoon coconut sugar

1 teaspoon vanilla extract

Pinch of sea salt

Preheat the oven to 375°F. In a large mixing bowl, mix together the flour, sugar, baking soda, spices, baking soda, and salt. In a separate mixing bowl, whisk together the egg, ghee, and vanilla. Fold the wet mixture into the dry mixture. Add the grated zucchini, carrot, apple, chopped dates, and walnuts. Mix together until fully combined.

Pour the mixture into a 12-cup muffin pan lined with paper muffin cups or greased with ghee. Bake for 20–25 minutes, until cooked through. Remove from the oven and allow to cool before serving. Enjoy with whipped cinnamon butter and a mug of hot chai.

While the bread bakes, prep the cinnamon butter. Combine all ingredients in a mixing bowl and cream together using a hand mixer. Taste and adjust flavorings as desired. Store in airtight container in the fridge for up to 5 days until ready to use.

DOSHA NOTES

Ⓟ Use flax eggs in place of eggs.

Ⓚ Skip the cinnamon butter.

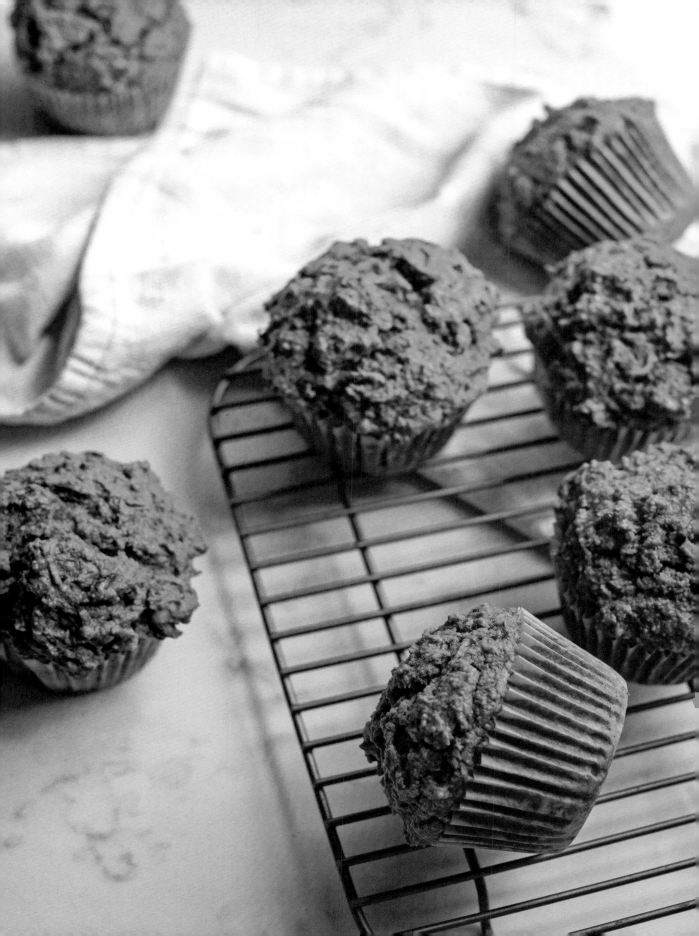

Chyawanprash Truffles

There's an Indian treat called *laddu* (or *ladoo*), made from sugar, flour, nuts or seeds, dried fruit, ground coconut, and spices. Each region has its own variation, but the roots of this treat are said to trace back to early Ayurvedic texts as a way to administer medicine. These little pistachio-rose truffles use dates as the base and sweetener, with a spoonful of chyawanprash, an herbal Ayurvedic jam with amalaki and herbs designed to boost your vitality in fall. The rejuvenating herbs and spices are wonderful for nourishing vata and pitta.

PREP: 2 minutes | COOK: 10 minutes | YIELD: 12 servings

TRUFFLES

1 cup unsalted pistachios

6 dates, pitted

1 tablespoon chyawanprash

1 teaspoon rose water

½ teaspoon vanilla extract

Pinch of ground cinnamon

Pinch of salt

FOR ROLLING

¼ cup finely shredded unsweetened coconut

2 tablespoons dried rose petals

½ teaspoon ground turmeric

Add the pistachios into a food processor and pulse until broken down into a fine pulp. Add the dates and pulse again. Add the remaining ingredients and pulse until the mixture starts to form into a ball. Taste and adjust flavors as desired. Roll into small 1-inch truffles. Place in the freezer to set for 10 minutes.

In a small bowl, mix together the coconut, rose petals, and turmeric. Roll each truffle in the mixture to coat. Store in the fridge in a sealed container up to a 5 days or until ready to eat.

DOSHA NOTES

Ⓚ Add ¼ teaspoon ground ginger; enjoy in moderation.

Ghee-Stuffed Dates

Quick little date snacks are my go-to treat when I want something sweet and simple. Ghee and dates are highly nourishing, ojas-boosting substances, while the sprinkle of salt helps balance the sweetness. If you're fighting holiday cravings, these date bites help satiate your sweet tooth without overburdening your system with processed sugar. Try tahini as an alternative to ghee inside these.

PREP: 2 minutes | YIELD: 4 servings

2 Medjool dates, pitted

½ teaspoon ghee

Pinch of sea salt

Slice the dates in half lengthwise and remove the pits. Stuff a tiny bit of ghee inside the pocket where the pit was and sprinkle salt on top.

Simple Stewed Apples

A simple stewed apple is a staple Ayurvedic recipe. When your digestive fire is low in the morning, this cooked apple breakfast can help jump-start agni. Substitute a pear for an alternative to the apple.

PREP: 5 minutes | COOK: 10 minutes | YIELD: 2 servings

2 cups water

2 apples, peeled, cored, and cut into ½-inch-thick slices

4 whole cloves

2 cardamom pods

1 cinnamon stick

In a small skillet, bring the water to a boil. Add the apples and spices, cover with a lid, and cook on medium heat for 8–10 minutes, until the apples are tender but not mushy. Drain the excess water. Enjoy warm on its own as a simple breakfast.

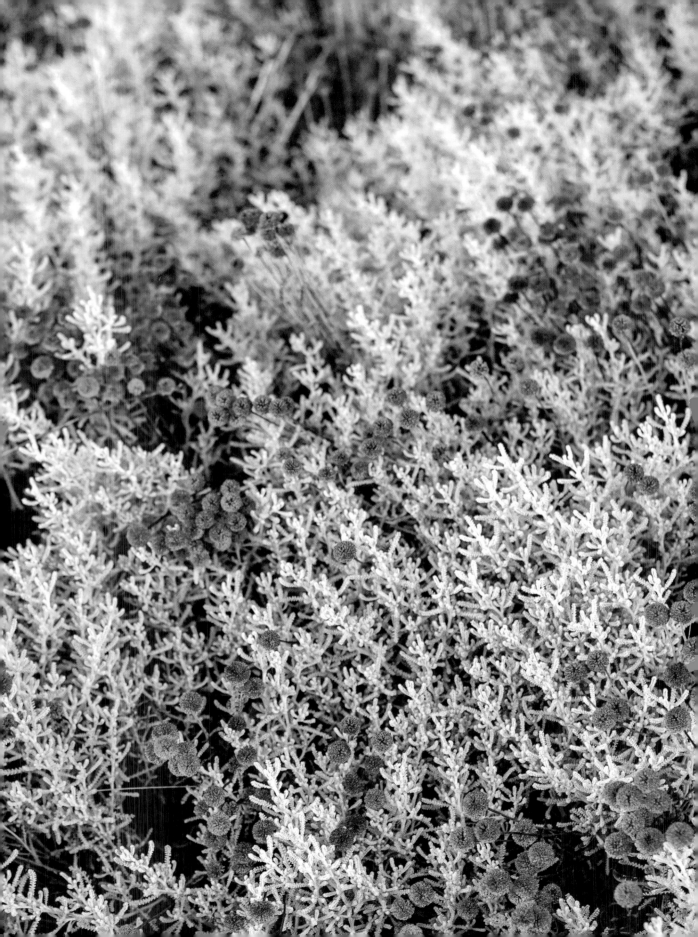

WINTER

Chilly frost. Windows fogged. Kettles on the stove. Winter brings quiet rest.

Winter straddles vata and kapha over the course of the season. In early winter, dry and cold weather bring increased vata. In late winter, wet and cold weather increase kapha. A winter seasonal practice requires you to pay close attention to how your environment shifts and how it influences you. You may need more oils, grounding foods, and slow practices in early winter, whereas more stimulating practices and foods will keep you from feeling stagnant as kapha increases toward spring. In this section, you'll find warming, grounding, and richer foods to stay balanced in the coldest months. If heavy, oily stews become too much in late winter, look toward the spring section to lighten up. With the dynamic changes that happen through the course of the season, it's even more important to stay present and aware of how you're feeling. This season's rituals offer a time for quiet inward reflection, encouraging more inward inquiry and dialogue.

Staying Balanced through Winter

EMPHASIZE

FOOD: Soupy, warm, and well-cooked meals of whole grains, legumes, root vegetables, cooked greens, and stewed fruits; pungent spices and healthy oils (ghee, sesame, sunflower); and quality dairy and animal proteins, if desired. Eat all meals in moderation and observe your digestive capacity.

BREATH: Invigorating, warming breathing that circulates energy through the body; Brahmari and Kapalbhati done at a steady pace; Nadi Shodhana to support the nervous system; deep and steady ujjayi breathing during asana to generate internal heat.

MOVEMENT: Warming, strengthening, and stabilizing practice with directed focus, moderate holds, and some repetition to break a sweat but not overexert yourself; sun salutations, heart openers, twists, forward folds, and inversions practiced in a warm environment are wonderful wintertime postures.

MEDITATION: Mantra repetition and kirtan, candle gazing (traṭaka), yoga nidra for deep rest.

MINIMIZE

FOOD: Raw vegetables; bitter and astringent foods; cold smoothies and iced drinks; ice cream and cold dairy; dried fruits and nuts; crackers, chips, and other dry snacking foods; overheating and grazing, especially on sugary treats or salty snacks.

BREATH: Cooling breathing, such as Sitali, or erratic and shallow breathing; absent breath awareness that leads to stagnation.

MOVEMENT: Fast and mobile activities, loud music or hyper-stimulating environments; lack of routine around exercise; becoming too sedentary or stagnant.

Tips for Tending Your Inner Fire in Winter

With the cold, heavy qualities of winter and richer foods, it's important to keep your agni burning bright. Try these tips for stoking your inner fire:

- Prepare a Ginger Appetizer (page 64) before each meal to kindle agni.

- Make lunch your main meal and enjoy lighter cooked meals at breakfast and dinner.

- Heavy sweets and cold ice cream can slow down digestion. Enjoy treats in moderation and in the daytime, instead of before bed.

- Take a short brisk walk after eating to avoid stagnation.

Winter Asana: *Nourishing*

In Patanjali's *Yoga Sutras*, yoga is described as the stilling of the restless mind. Asana and pranayama ultimately lead us to a place of stillness, an experience of our true nature beyond the fluctuations of thought and attachments to identity. When was the last time you deeply rested? Winter is a time to honor the natural stilling of the outer world and give ourselves permission for a sacred pause to replenish. In early winter, try this practice by moving slowly. Instead of racing through the sun salutations, move with intention and steady breath to soothe and stabilize vata. Toward late winter, you may pick up the pace to break a sweat, build more heat, and move you out of the winter blues to balance kapha. As you move through this practice, ask yourself, "What does deep nourishment feel like in my body? How can I invite more joy into my life?"

WINTER PRACTICE TIPS

- Focus on warmth, stability, ease, and inward reflection.

- Practice steady ujjayi breathing to warm your body.

- Practice with a moderate pace to generate heat, but avoid overworking yourself.

- Slow down when needed.

DOSHA NOTES

Ⓥ Practice at a steady pace with focus on even breathing and stability in the postures, never overextending or tiring yourself out.

Ⓟ Move at a moderate pace and maintain an attitude of lightness.

Ⓚ Emphasize deep breathing, longer holds, and fluid movements that build heat and strength.

SURYA NAMASKAR (SUN SALUTATION SEQUENCE)

Start this sequence with 3–5 rounds of Surya Namaskar (page 83). A winter Surya Namaskar can be practiced at a steady pace to produce heat but never too much to overextend or exhaust yourself. Emphasize long, even inhalations and exhalations timed with each movement.

VASISTHASANA (SIDE PLANK POSE)

Begin in a plank position. Walk your feet together, squeeze your inner thighs, and engage your glutes. Shift weight into your right hand and rotate your body to face the left side of the mat. Extend your left arm toward the sky. Hold for 5 breaths. Repeat on the other side.

MODIFICATIONS

• Lower your bottom knee to the ground for support.

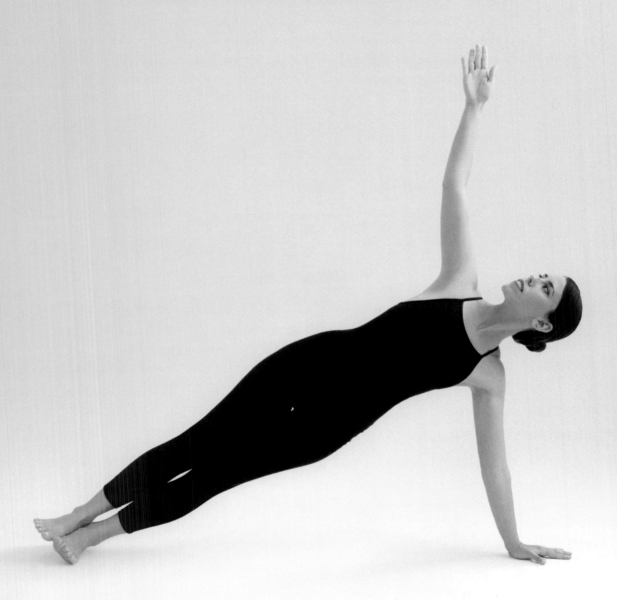

PARIVRTTA UTKATASANA (TWISTED CHAIR POSE)

From standing, step both feet together with big toes touching and heels slightly apart. Inhale, draw your hands together in prayer position at the center of your chest. Exhale, bend your knees and sit back like you're sitting in a chair. Lift your upper body and broaden your chest. Inhale, lengthen your spine. Exhale, twist right around your navel and lower your elbow to the outside of your right thigh. Hold for 5 breaths. Repeat on the other side. Return to standing when done.

MODIFICATIONS

- Place a block between your thighs with feet hip-distance apart for more stability.

- Keep your torso upright and twist gently.

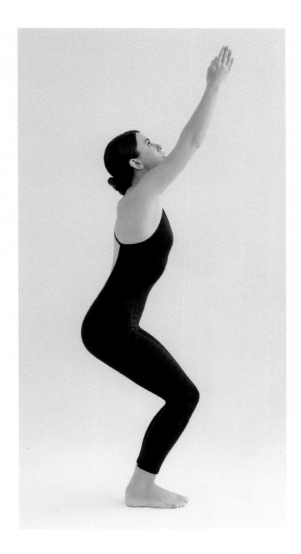 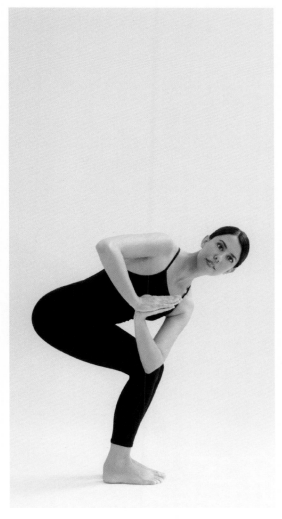

TRIKONASANA (TRIANGLE POSE)

From standing, step your feet as wide as your arms reach and rotate your body to face the side of the mat. Turn your right foot forward and keep your left foot facing to the side. Inhale, engage your quadriceps and lengthen your spine. Exhale, reach forward over your right leg and extend your upper body parallel to the floor. Rotate your arms perpendicular to the floor, press the back of your right hand into your calf and extend your left arm overhead. Gaze toward the top hand. Hold for 5 breaths. Repeat on the other side.

MODIFICATIONS

- Use a block or chair to support the lower hand for balance and support.

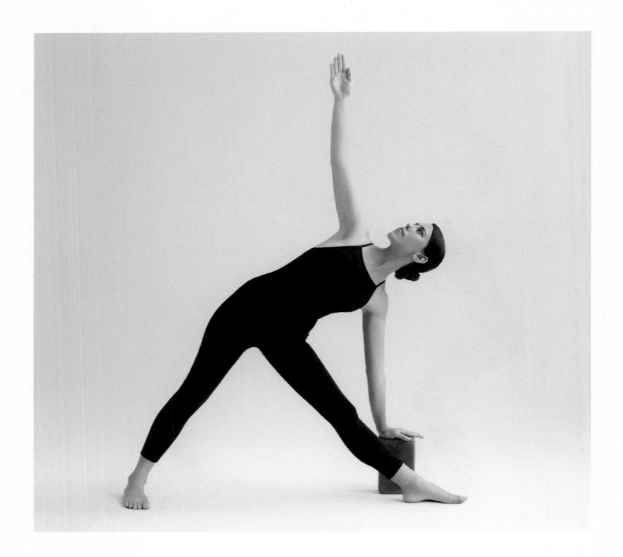

UTTHITA HASTA PADANGUSTASANA
(EXTENDED HAND-TO-BIG-TOE POSE)

From standing, shift weight onto your right leg to balance. Draw your left knee into your chest. Hold here or wrap your index and middle fingers around left big toe and straighten your leg. Hold for 5 breaths. Repeat on the other side.

MODIFICATIONS

- Use a wall for stability.

- For tight hamstrings, keep your knee bent and focus on balance.

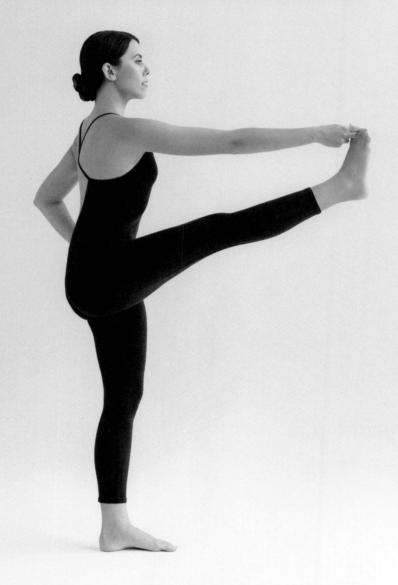

NATARAJASANA (KING DANCER POSE)

From standing, balance on your left leg. Bend your right knee and draw your heel to your right buttock. Reach back with the right hand, palm facing outward, and grab the inside of your right foot or ankle. Stay here to work on balance or continue to the full extension of the pose. Inhale, extend your left arm overhead. Exhale, press your foot into your hand and lift your leg away from the ground. Arch your upper back and lean forward, reaching outward with your left hand and kicking into your left leg in opposition, to balance. Hold for 5 breaths. Repeat on the other side.

MODIFICATIONS

- Use a wall for stability.

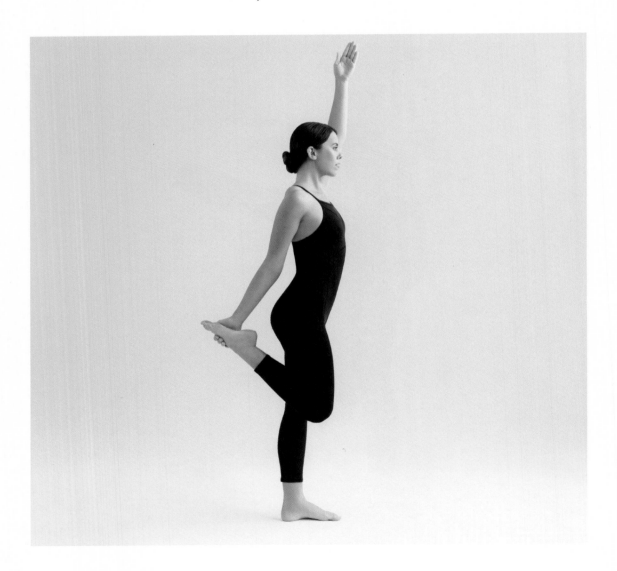

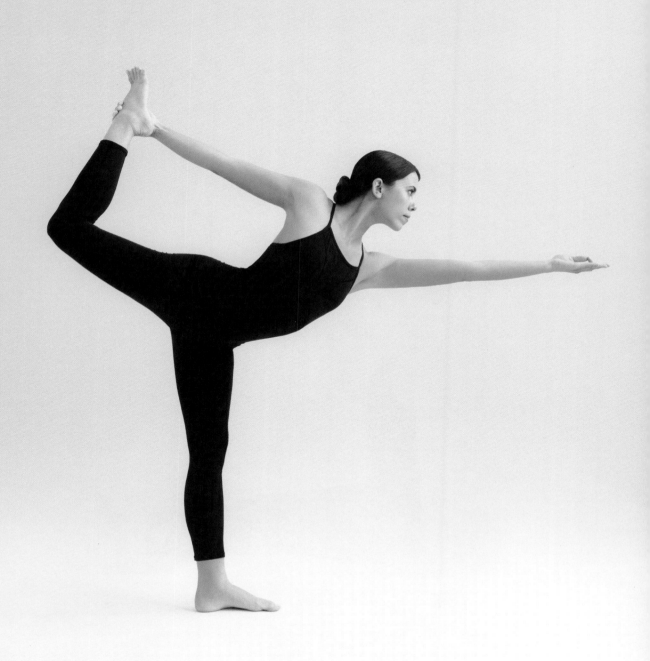

DANDASANA (STAFF POSE)

Sit upright with your legs extended straight in front of you. Inhale, extend your spine and place your palms flat by your hips with your fingers pointing forward. Exhale, lengthen the back of your neck and draw your chin toward your chest. Hold for 5 breaths. Release and repeat 1–2 more times.

MODIFICATIONS
• Elevate your hips with a folded blanket.

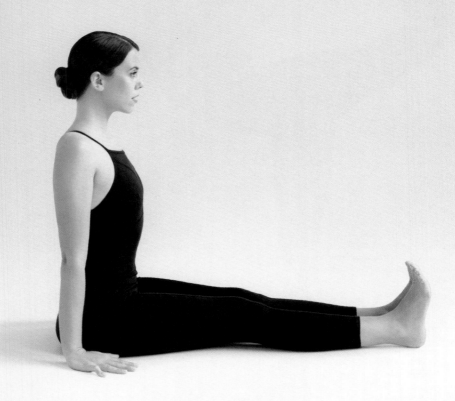

PURVOTTANASANA (UPWARD PLANK POSE)

Sit upright with your legs extended straight in front of you. Inhale, extend your spine and place your palms 12 inches behind your hips with your fingers pointing forward. Exhale, bend your elbows. Inhale, lift your hips and shoulders in a straight line and press the bottoms of your feet to the ground. Keep your neck in line with your spine and avoid dropping your head back and pinching your neck. Hold for 5 breaths. Lower your hips and return to seated.

MODIFICATIONS
- Bend your knees for a reverse tabletop position to lessen strain on your back.

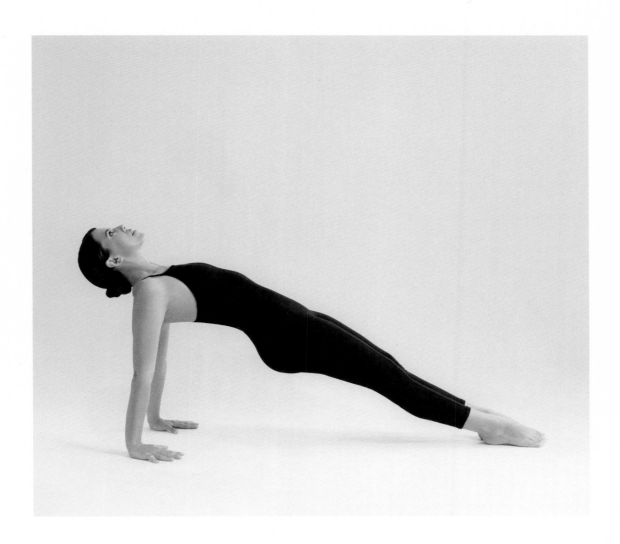

EKA PADA RAJAKAPOTASANA (PIGEON POSE)

Begin on your hands and knees, draw your right knee forward behind your right hand with your shin on the ground and your right foot angled back toward your left hip. If your right hip is off the ground, use a folded blanket or pillow underneath your hip for support. Extend your left leg straight behind you and lower your hips to the ground. Uncurl your back toes to rest on the top of the foot. Keep your hips level. Place your hands by your hips or slightly in front of your legs. Hold for 5–10 breaths.

MODIFICATIONS
- Lie on your back and bend your knees with feet on the floor. Cross your one ankle above the opposite knee and draw your legs to the chest.

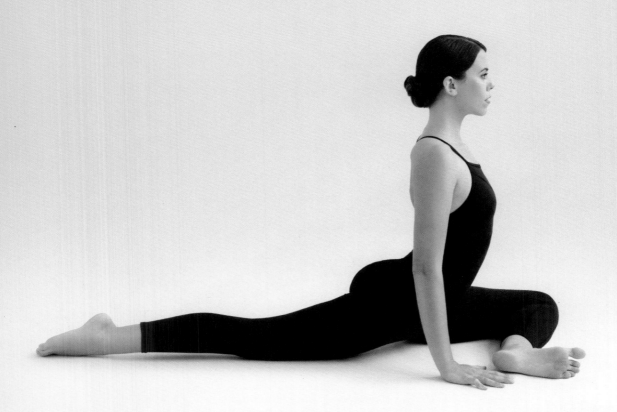

GOMUKHASANA (COW FACE POSE)

Sit upright with your legs extended straight in front of you. Bend both knees and put your feet on the floor. Cross your legs, stacking your right knee on top of your left with both feet pointed back by your hips. Inhale, reach your right arm toward the sky and internally rotate your arm. Exhale, bend your elbow and place your right palm between your shoulder blades. Inhale, reach your left arm out to the side and internally rotate your arm. Exhale, reach behind your back and place the back of the left hand on your upper back, reaching both hands toward each other to clasp fingers. Roll your shoulders open and lift your heart. Hold for 5 breaths. Gently release. Repeat on the other side.

MODIFICATIONS

- Try this with one leg crossed and one leg extended straight to lessen strain on your knees.

- Use a strap between your hands to hold on to and focus on shoulder opening.

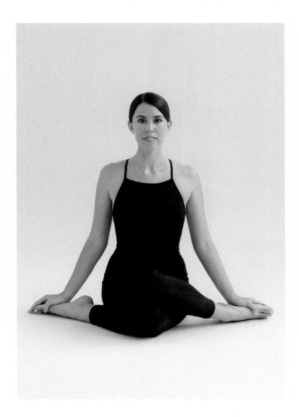
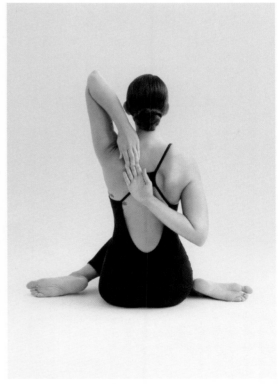

VIPARITA KARANI (LEGS AGAINST THE WALL POSE)

Place a folded blanket, pillow, or bolster at a wall. Sit down with your hip at the wall and lie down on your back. Extend your legs up the wall. Lift your hips and slide the support under your pelvis and low back, elevating your hips above your heart. Hold for 5–10 minutes.

MODIFICATIONS

- Place a bolster, pillow, or folded blanket under your hips for elevation or under your neck for additional support.

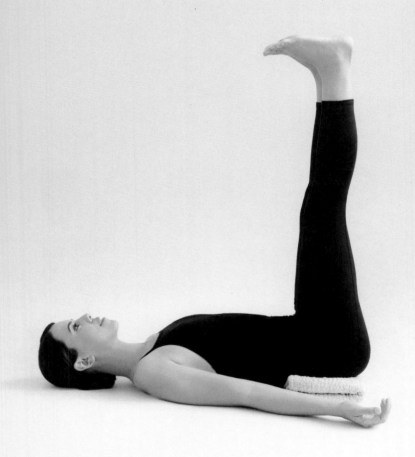

SAVASANA (CORPSE POSE)

The queen of all poses—do not skip this one! Set a gentle alarm if you're worried you may fall asleep. Lie on your back with your legs extended long and your palms resting by your sides. Cover yourself with a blanket and support your joints by placing a pillow or bolster behind your knees. Cover your eyes with an eye pillow or cloth. Close your eyes, exhale deeply, and relax every inch of your body. Release any controlled effort to breathe. Rest in stillness for 7–15 minutes to complete your practice.

MODIFICATIONS
- Place an extra folded blanket or sandbag on your pelvis for weight, for grounding.

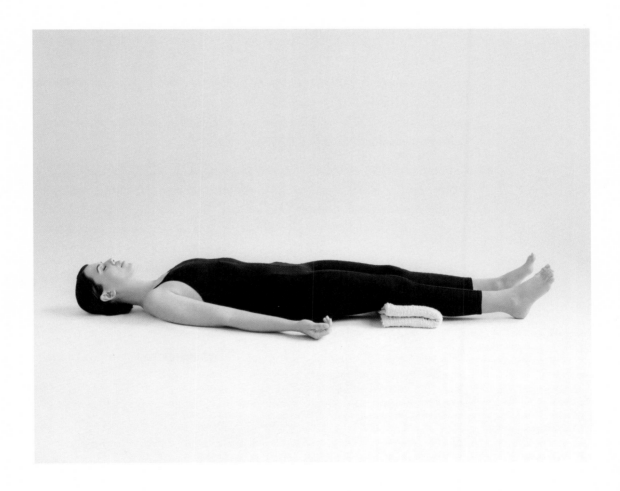

Winter Pranayama: *Bhramari*

This is one of my favorite breath practices for the sheer amount of joy it brings! *Bhram* in Sanskrit means "bee," thus this pranayama gets its name from the buzzing sound produced during the exhale, the "resonant hum of inner consciousness," as Vedic teacher and author Bri Maya Tiwari describes. What makes this practice unique is the act of withdrawing the senses by closing off your ears, eyes, and mouth with a gesture of your hands known as *shanmukhi mudra*. This withdrawal of external sensory stimulation allows us to rest in an experience of inner stillness. Winter's quiet, internal nature gives us opportunity to withdraw and look within ourselves.

HOW TO

In the humming of this breath, the vibration of your vocal cords stimulate your thyroid and pineal and pituitary glands, soothing your nervous system and releasing cerebral tension. The result is an elated, clear state in your mind and freedom from the constant internal chatter. It's important to practice Bhramari sitting upright, and it's most potent when done in the early morning hours.

1   Sit in a comfortable upright position that supports your spine and hips. This can be done cross-legged on the floor or seated in a chair. However you choose to sit, make sure your hips are relaxed and your head, neck, and spine are aligned. Relax your shoulders, neck, and jaw. Soften your belly.

2   Lift both hands to your face and gently rest your index fingers on your closed eyelids with the lightest pressure. Place your middle fingers on either side of your nose, where the bone meets the cartilage. Place your ring fingers on your upper lip and your pinkies below your bottom lip. Use gentle pressure to hold your lips closed. Last, use your thumbs to gently close your ears by lightly pressing on the tragus, the small flap in front of your ear canal. This hand position forms shanmukhi mudra. If shanmukhi mudra feels overwhelming, you can simply plug your ears with your thumbs and gently rest the palms of your hands over your closed eyes.

3   With gates of perception closed, draw your inner attention to your third eye, the space between your brows on your forehead.

4   Take a deep breath in through both nostrils and down into your belly, and place the tip of your tongue on your soft palate. As you exhale, make a humming "mmmm" sound with your mouth closed. You'll feel a vibration in your upper palate, teeth, and throat. Contract your belly to elongate the sound on the exhale.

5   Repeat 5–10 times, focusing on making the quality of the breath and sound feel smooth and steady.

6   When complete, rest your hands in your lap with your eyes closed. Notice the subtle vibrations reverberating through your body. Notice the stillness of your mind. Sit quietly for another 5–10 minutes to integrate the experience.

PRACTICE NOTE

This breath meditation is generally safe for everyone. However, if you have epilepsy or an active ear infection, it's best to practice this without a mudra and simply feel the vibration of the humming with your eyes open in a soft, resting gaze.

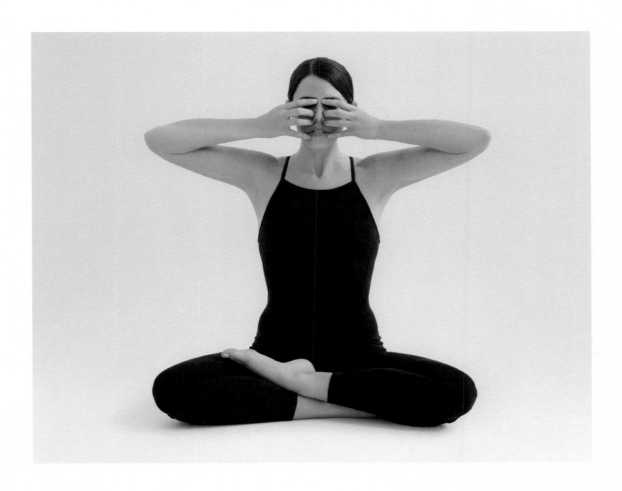

Winter Lunar Ritual: *Waning Moon*

From the full moon to the new moon, the period when the moon grows darker is the waning moon phase of the lunar cycle. This phase signals a time of lessening and letting go. It's a time for organizing and making space for the quiet, contemplative time around the new moon. Rather than looking to ways you can improve your life with a new diet or a lifestyle change, this ritual asks you first to look at what needs to be cut away in order to free up more energy in your life.

WOMEN'S LUNAR RITUAL

The waning moon aligns with the luteal phase. Estrogen has peaked and now progesterone is on the rise. Dr. Christiane Northrup shares, "The luteal phase, from ovulation until the onset of menstruation, is when women are most in tune with their inner knowing and with what isn't working in their lives." You might feel more inspired to organize, close loops on projects, and begin to prepare for rest. Moving toward an increasing vata, you may feel bloated or have slower digestion. Belly breathing, abdominal massage, castor oil packs, and gentle movement can help you stay balanced leading up to menstruation.

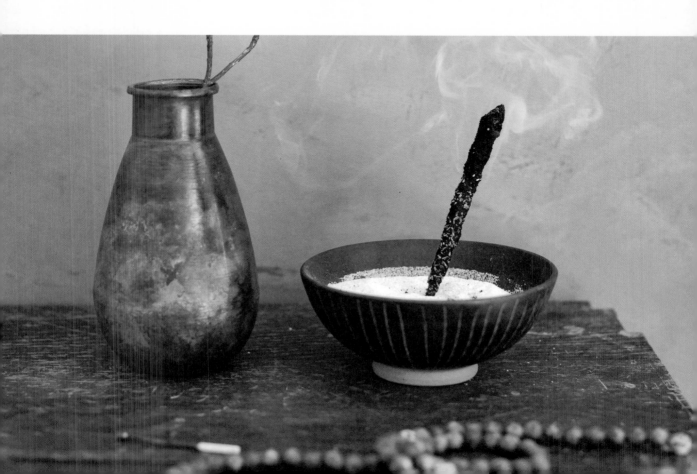

THE ELEVENTH-DAY FAST

I remember sitting at a cafe in college and overhearing two men talking about how incredible one felt after fasting on the eleventh day. I made a note in my phone: "fasting, moon, eleventh day." Years later, as I started to study yoga and Ayurveda, this little clue I'd written down finally came to life.

Known as Ekadasi in the Vedic tradition, the eleventh day after the full or new moon is an optimal time for fasting. While winter is not particularly a recommended time for deep cleansing or extended fasting, a simple single-day fast can do wonders for rebooting your body and mind. Especially if your digestive fire is low or you need a reset around the holidays, taking a day or two a month to fast can have powerful transformative effects in your life. Eating lightly helps increase digestive fire, which in turn helps increase overall energy and clarity. But note here that fasting doesn't necessarily have to mean food. You can also fast from media, talking, or anything that is engaging and mentally stimulating. This lunar fast can also go hand in hand with a silent retreat.

THE RITUAL

Mark your calendars for the eleventh day after the full moon. In this waning moon time, when your energy is naturally lower and so is your agni, plan a day of rest to recalibrate your inner fire. Eat lightly in the morning, fasting or enjoying a small bowl of Simple Stewed Apples (page 243) for breakfast; try the Simple Mung Soup (page 278) or Immunity Broth (page 223) for lunch and dinner. Sip on Warming Agni Tea (page 272) and CCF Tea (page 65) throughout the day.

Fasting has a long tradition in spiritual lineages to bring us closer to the divine and seeing ourselves more clearly. It helps to quiet the inner chatter and clear the fog of our minds. With the clarity that comes from fasting, explore the following questions in contemplation and journaling:

- Do my daily activities nourish me?

- Am I using my energy effectively and efficiently?

- Are there areas of my life that could use more attention?

- What am I ready to let go of to create more space in my life?

Winter Seasonal Ritual: *Solstice Silent Retreat*

In winter, the earth sleeps in stillness. As the sun slips into the most southern point, there is a momentary pause, a suspension between the solar inhalation and exhalation. Winter solstice brings the end of the year's solar cycle and an opportunity for a sacred pause in our own lives to welcome stillness and inward reflection. There is a clear turning point in all cycles, a momentary opportunity to embrace this ephemeral state between fullness and emptiness. Solstice is this time—the time to honor all that we have cultivated in this past year, integrate lessons, and look to where space can be created in our lives in the year ahead.

The mind needs solitude in order to digest life's experiences. Silence is also the simplest remedy for balancing vata dosha. When we've talked too much, traveled too much, or feel overstimulated by life's constant sensory input, a retreat is a necessary friend on our path. As you plan your retreat, let me first give a disclaimer.

For me, stillness is not necessarily comfortable or even enjoyable in the beginning. It's important to note that while a retreat sounds luxurious, it actually can stir some feelings of discomfort. And that's perfectly okay. You might find yourself wanting to reach for your phone, feeling phantom scrolling pains or the sense of anxiety that you're not accomplishing enough. Those feelings might not fade right away, and that's perfectly okay. We tend to have this romanticized picture in our minds of what meditating should look and feel like. But what is rarely pictured is the internal struggle we face of needing to feel productive while also desiring to feel that stillness within. Like anything, it's a practice. You don't start lifting weights with a 50-pound dumbbell. You start with 5-pound weights and build the strength over time. Do your best to enter this retreat space without expectation or desire to accomplish anything by the end. The goal is to create spaciousness to simply be. After all, isn't that who are? Human beings—not human doings.

I give an outline for a daylong silent solstice retreat at home. However, this is a very personal practice and can be adjusted to meet your needs. If you have kids, this may be an early morning of silence to yourself, or an afternoon, if you have a sitter. Whatever the time slot, the intention is to create spaciousness to be with yourself, free of distractions. Set your away responders and tell your friends and family of your plans of your inward journey. Take care of your most pressing to-dos in preparation for this time and leave the rest out of the ritual.

THE RITUAL

- Wake before the sun, between 5 and 7 a.m. These predawn hours, Brahmamuhurta, is prized in Ayurveda as the "ambrosial hours," where nature supports this sense of inner quietude and where meditation is most easily supported. If you have kids, this is also a crucial time to get a moment to yourself before your family wakes.

- Cleanse your senses by following your dinacharya routine. Do this in silence and with an inward focus. It's easy to quickly become overstimulated moving around the house. Try to keep your focus to your morning body care before meditation.

- Before eating, sit down in your practice space for meditation and reflection. Light a candle and offer some flowers or fresh fruit on your altar. Close your eyes and spend 5–30 minutes in meditation.

- Continue on to movement. Try the Nourishing Winter Yoga Sequence (page 247) and end with 10 rounds of Bhramari pranayama (page 260), observing the contrast of silence and sound in this meditation.

- Spend the rest of your planned time in silence. Avoid talking, texting, emailing, or any kind of communication with the outer world.

- Keep a journal during your retreat. Write down any feelings and thoughts as they arise. Where do you feel resistance to the experience? What is needed to feel more ease?

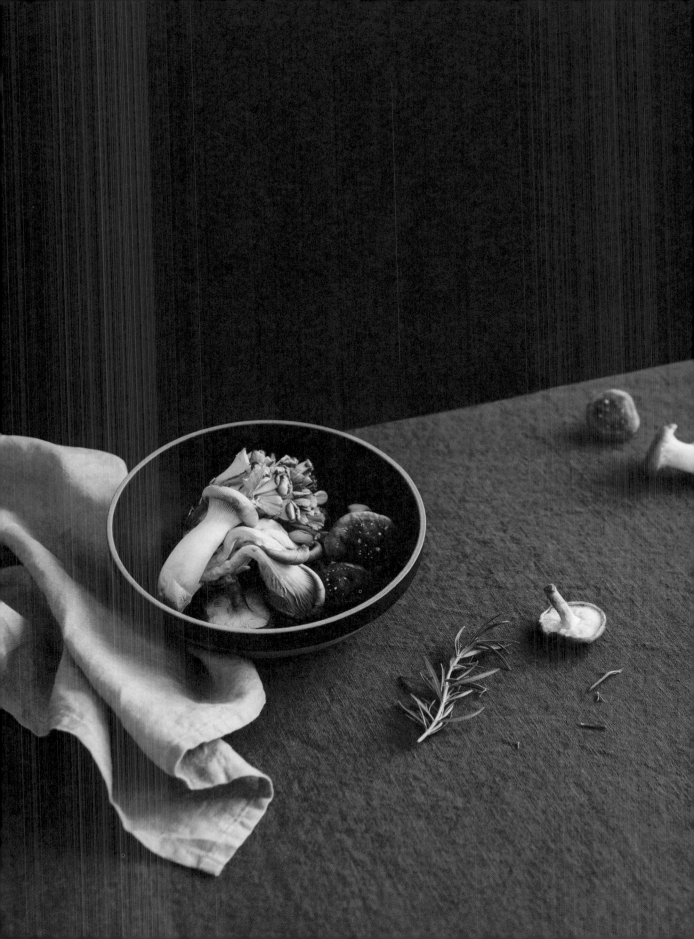

Winter Recipes

Drinks

Breakfast

Soups, Salads & Sides

Main Dishes

Sweet

Black Sesame Latte

Here is a mineral-rich coffee alternative to satisfy your morning hot beverage ritual. Black sesame seeds are rich in healthy fats and supportive for the kidneys. Sesame is also heating, making the oil, seed, and paste a good option for cold-weather months. I like to make a jar of fresh black sesame paste in advance to have on hand for a quick creamy coffee-free morning latte.

PREP: 20 minutes | COOK: 5 minutes | YIELD: 2 servings

BLACK SESAME PASTE

1 cup black sesame seeds

¼ cup untoasted sesame oil

LATTE

2 cups milk (organic raw dairy milk or nondairy milk of choice)

2 tablespoons black sesame paste

1 tablespoon raw honey

In a large skillet on low heat, toast the black sesame seeds for 1–2 minutes. Stir frequently to avoid burning. Because these are black, it can be difficult to see if they're burning, so it's best to stay with them the whole time they're on the stove. Transfer the toasted seeds to a high-speed blender or food processor. Add the sesame oil and blend until creamy. You may have to stop and scrape the sides several times until it is fully incorporated. Add more oil to loosen the mixture as needed. Store in an airtight jar in fridge for up to a month and use as needed.

In a high-speed blender, combine the milk and black sesame paste. Blend until creamy. Strain through a nut milk bag or cheesecloth for a smoother texture. Transfer the strained milk to a small pot and heat on low heat. Once hot, pour back into the blender, add the raw honey, and blend on high until frothy. Pour into a mug and enjoy hot.

DOSHA NOTES

Ⓟ Use maple syrup instead of honey.

Ⓚ Try this recipe with almond milk.

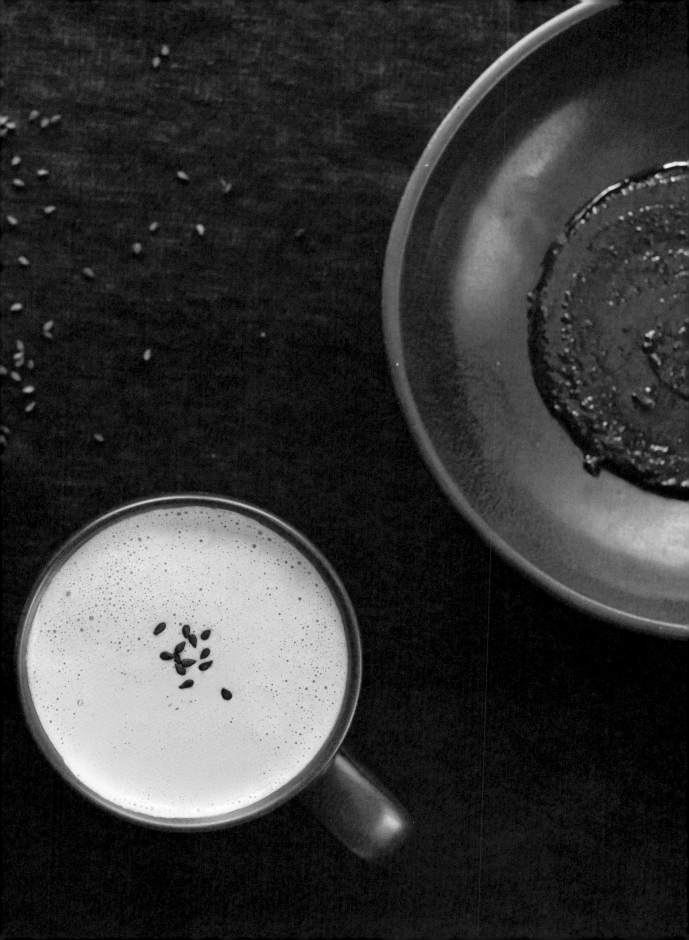

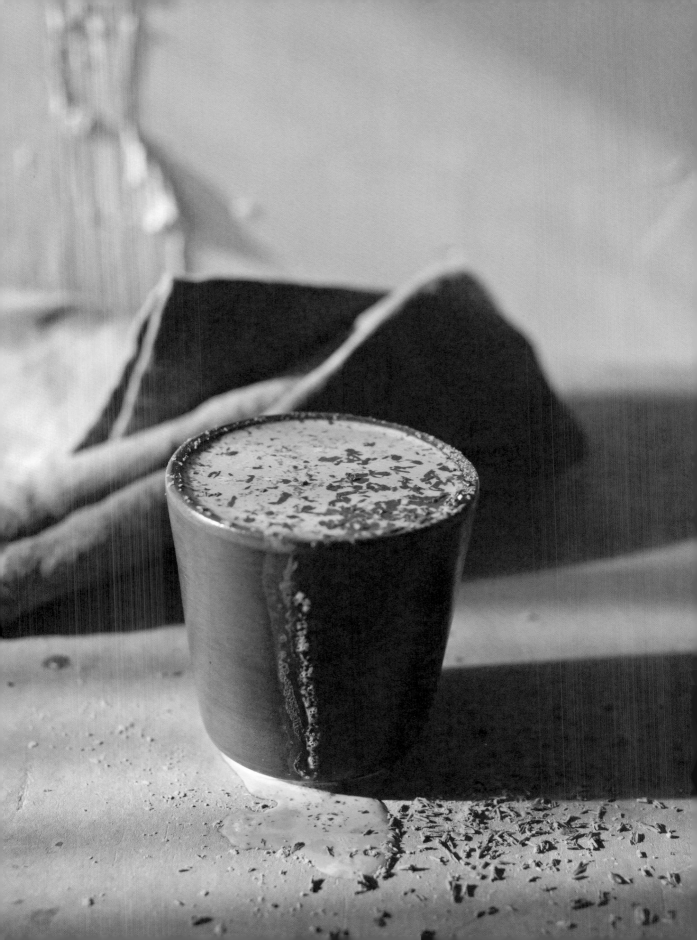

Chai Hot Chocolate

Hot chocolate is the ultimate comforting winter drink. But chocolate can be quite drying and aggravating to vata dosha. Try raw cacao powder with a pinch of cardamom and ghee to reduce the stimulating effects. I also make this drink with carob powder in place of the cacao. Carob is a more sattvic alternative to chocolate that has a similar rich and earthy flavor.

PREP: 5 minutes | COOK: 2 minutes | YIELD: 1–2 servings

2 cups hot milk (organic raw dairy milk or nondairy milk of choice)

2–3 tablespoons raw cacao powder or carob powder

1 tablespoon maple syrup

1 teaspoon ghee

¼ teaspoon ground cardamom

¼ teaspoon ground cinnamon

Pinch of ground clove

In a small pot, heat the milk on low heat to bring just under a boil. Transfer to a high-speed blender and add the remaining ingredients. Blend until creamy. Pour into a mug and enjoy hot.

DOSHA NOTES

(P) Swap cacao for carob powder.

(K) Omit ghee.

Orange Peel & Licorice Tea

Licorice root is known for its ability to nourish the adrenals, support the lungs, and soothe the throat. In deep winter, this simple sattvic tea provides warming comfort and balance for both vata and kapha doshas.

PREP: 2 minutes | COOK: 10 minutes | YIELD: 4 servings

4 cups water

Peel of 1 fresh organic orange, roughly chopped, or 2 tablespoons dried orange peel

1 tablespoon dried cut licorice root

Optional: 1 teaspoon raw honey

In a small pot, bring water to a boil. Add in the orange peel and licorice root. Simmer on medium heat for 5 minutes. Turn off heat, cover, and steep for another 5 minutes. Strain the liquid and discard the pulp. For a little extra sweetness, stir in a spoonful of raw honey at the end. Serve hot.

Note: When using peel or zest, always opt for organic. Conventional citrus rinds can hold toxic chemicals and might be covered in waxes or injected with dyes.

Warming Agni Tea

In cold winter months, when the fire element is low our bodies need a little extra support to boost our internal fire. This digestive tea with ginger and cayenne helps bring heat back to the belly and increases agni.

PREP: 2 minutes | COOK: 10 minutes | YIELD: 4 servings 4 cups water

2 tablespoons roughly chopped fresh ginger

1 tablespoon lemon or lime juice

1 teaspoon raw honey

Small pinch of cayenne

In a small pot, bring water to a boil. Add the ginger and simmer on medium heat for 5 minutes. Turn off heat, cover, and steep for another 5 minutes. Strain the liquid and discard the pulp. Stir in the lemon juice, raw honey, and cayenne. Sip hot between meals.

DOSHA NOTES

(P) Skip this tea if overheated.

Golden Milk Oats

This oatmeal recipe is anything but boring. Taking cues from the classic golden milk drink, these oats are well spiced with warming turmeric, ginger, cardamom, and cinnamon for an extra punch to your morning porridge. If oats leave you feeling tired or heavy, try cracked buckwheat or brown rice farina as an alternative.

PREP: 5 minutes | COOK: 10 minutes | YIELD: 2 servings

2 cups water

½ inch fresh ginger, minced or ½ teaspoon ground ginger

½ inch fresh turmeric, minced or 1 teaspoon ground turmeric

1 cup gluten-free rolled oats

½ cup raisins

½ teaspoon ground cinnamon

¼ teaspoon ground cardamom

Pinch of salt

Optional: 1 teaspoon ghee, splash of milk, 1 tablespoon maple syrup

In a small pot, bring water to a boil on high heat. Add the ginger and turmeric (see note) and steep for 2–3 minutes. Once the water turns a golden color, stir in the oats and reduce heat to medium-low. The secret to cooking oats is not to stir the pot. Cover and cook for 7–10 minutes, until liquid is almost fully absorbed. Add the raisins and remove from heat. Stir in the remaining spices and salt. Divide between bowls to serve. Top with a spoonful of ghee, splash of milk, and a drizzle of maple syrup, if desired.

Note: If you're using ground ginger and turmeric instead of fresh, skip the first step of steeping the roots and add in with the other ground spices at the end.

DOSHA NOTES
Ⓟ Omit ginger.
Ⓚ Try with cracked buckwheat in place of oats.

Carrot Cake Pancakes with Labneh Frosting

As the name states, these pancakes taste like carrot cake and are a special breakfast treat I like to serve around the winter holidays. Fresh grated carrot brings texture and nutrients to this mix, while digestive-boosting spices give these pancakes a rich taste. Labneh is a cultured yogurt with a lightly sour taste that works great as a healthy alternative to cream cheese frosting. Substitute Greek yogurt or a thick coconut yogurt if you can't find labneh.

PREP: 15 minutes | COOK: 30 minutes | YIELD: 4 servings

PANCAKES

2 cups organic pancake flour mix of your choice

1 teaspoon ground cinnamon

½ teaspoon ground nutmeg

½ teaspoon ground ginger

¼ teaspoon salt

1 cup grated carrot (about 1 large carrot)

½ cup unsweetened raisins

1½ cups almond milk

1 egg

2 tablespoons maple syrup, plus more for serving

2 tablespoons orange juice

1 tablespoon orange zest

2 tablespoons pistachios, roughly chopped

2–3 teaspoon ghee or coconut oil, for frying

LABNEH FROSTING

½ cup organic labneh or plain fresh Greek yogurt

1 tablespoon maple syrup

1 teaspoon orange zest

Optional: 1 teaspoon orange blossom water

In a large mixing bowl, combine the pancake flour mix, spices, and salt. Add the grated carrots and raisins to the dry mixture. In a separate bowl, whisk together the milk, egg, maple syrup, orange juice, and orange zest. Fold the wet mixture into the dry until fully incorporated.

Preheat the oven to 200°F to keep the pancakes warm. To cook, warm a griddle or skillet on medium heat to start, once hot reduce to medium-low heat. Melt a dab of ghee or coconut oil, then pour about ¼ cup of batter into the pan for each pancake. Keep the heat low to cook slowly until the pancake is golden on one side, then flip and cook until golden on the other side. Place the finished pancakes on baking sheet in the oven to keep warm while cooking the rest. Repeat until you've worked through all batter. Serve hot with a spoonful of labneh frosting, a sprinkle of chopped pistachios, and a drizzle of warm maple syrup.

For the frosting: Combine all ingredients in a small bowl and mix together. Taste and adjust seasonings as desired. This is best made fresh before serving.

DOSHA NOTES

Ⓟ Omit ground ginger.

Ⓚ Omit egg; use 2 tablespoons ground flax in ¼ cup water instead.

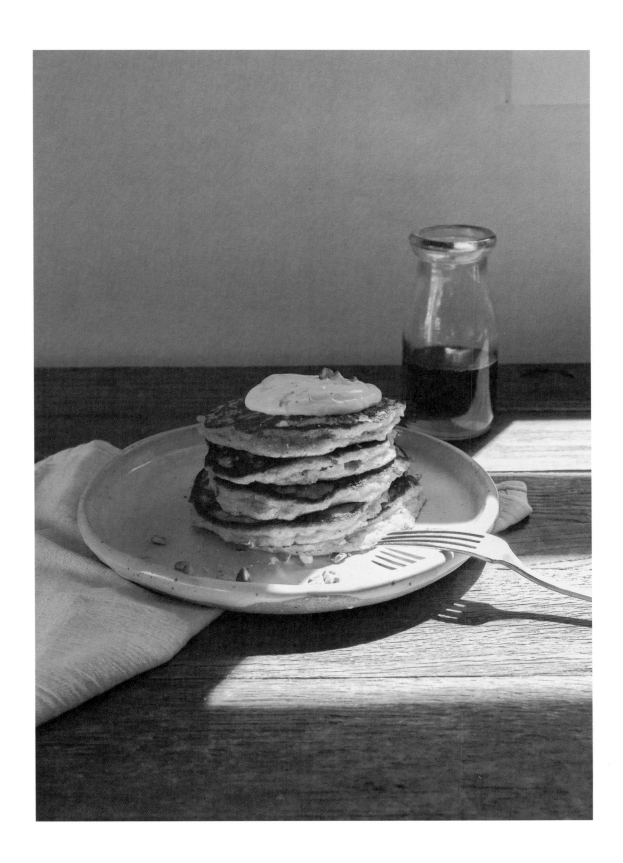

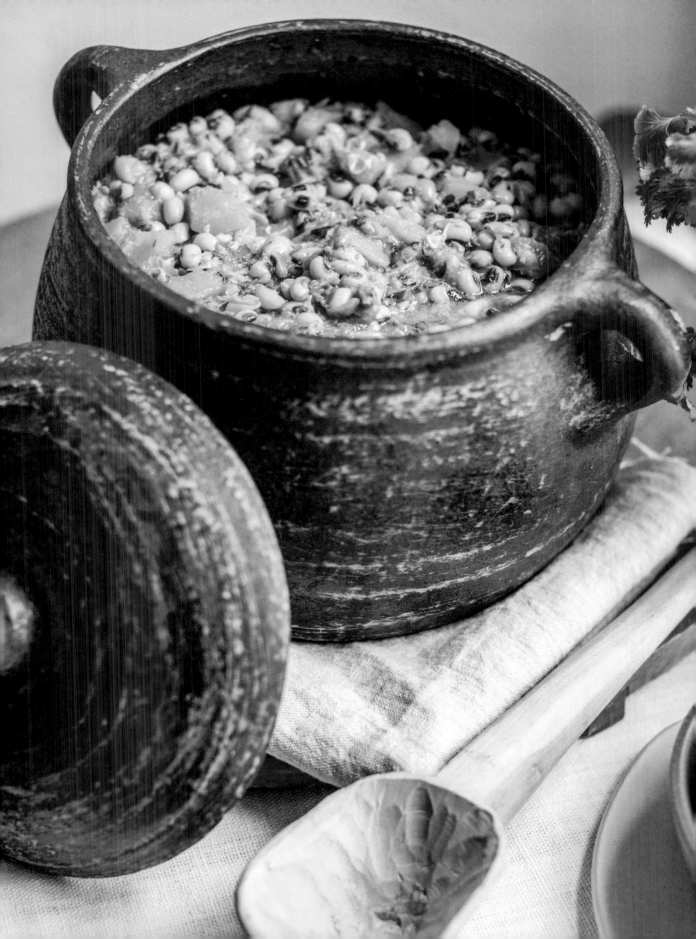

Black-Eyed Pea & Pumpkin Stew

What makes this simple winter stew interesting is the unexpected addition of rose hips, which are not commonly used in the kitchen. My friend Robin introduced these to me as an alternative to tomatoes in savory cooked dishes. Since canned tomatoes can be acidic and difficult to digest, rose hips offer an alternative with a vibrant tart flavor to a dish while providing a boost of extra vitamin C. Try grinding rose hips in a coffee grinder or blender for an easy homemade rose hip powder.

PREP: 20 minutes, plus 8–12 hours for soaking | COOK: 50 minutes | YIELD: 4 servings

1 tablespoon dried cut rosehips

3 tablespoons ghee or olive oil

½ cup leeks, finely chopped

2 tablespoons minced or grated fresh ginger

1 tablespoon mustard seeds

1 tablespoon cumin seeds

1 teaspoon ground coriander

¼ teaspoon ground cinnamon

1 cup dried black-eyed peas, soaked overnight (3 cups soaked)

4 cups cubed pumpkin or butternut squash

6–7 cups water

1 teaspoon salt

½ cup roughly chopped cilantro

1–2 tablespoons fresh lime juice

To make the rose hip powder, grind rose hips in a clean coffee grinder or a high-speed blender until it makes a fine powder.

In a large pot, heat the ghee on medium heat and stir in the leeks and ginger. Sauté for 1–2 minutes, until tender. Add the mustard seeds, cumin seeds, coriander, and cinnamon. Mix in the beans and pumpkin, stirring to coat in the spices. Add the water, rosehip powder, and salt. Bring to a boil, cover with a lid, and simmer for 30 minutes on medium heat. Reduce heat to low and cook for another 20 minutes, until the beans are tender and the water is absorbed, to make a thick stew. Stir in the cilantro and lime juice. Taste and adjust seasonings. Serve hot.

DOSHA NOTES
Ⓟ Omit mustard seeds.
Ⓚ Reduce ghee.

Simple Mung Soup

When your digestion is sluggish or your energy is low, this simple mung soup is a wonderful cleansing recipe to rekindle your inner fire. Make this soup as a fasting dish when you're taking a day in silence to rest your body and mind. Don't be fooled by the simplicity of the ingredients list—this soup is surprisingly satiating and packed with flavor.

PREP: 8–12 hours for soaking | COOK: 40 minutes | Serving: 4 servings

¼ cup dry whole mung beans

5 cups water, plus more for soaking mung beans

2 inches fresh ginger, minced

1 teaspoon ghee

¼ teaspoon salt

¼ cup cilantro, chopped

Place the dry mung beans in a large bowl, cover with water, and soak overnight. Drain and rinse well the next day. Don't skip this step; it's essential for a quicker cook time and an easier-to-digest meal.

In a medium pot, bring 5 cups water to a boil. Add the soaked mung beans, ginger, ghee, and salt. Cover with a lid and simmer on medium heat for 45 minutes. Remove from heat, stir in the cilantro, and enjoy hot.

DOSHA NOTES

Ⓥ Increase to 1 tablespoon ghee.

Ⓟ Reduce ginger.

Braised Winter Greens

Raw greens can be difficult to digest, especially in winter and for vata and kapha types. Braising greens in a hot pan with spices is a wonderful way to increase their digestibility and add a punch of flavor. Cooking them reduces their bitter tastes and increases their sweetness, making greens more balancing and easier to digest. Try this method with a variety of different greens and spices through the seasons.

PREP: 5 minutes | COOK: 5 minutes | YIELD: 4 servings

1 bunch collard greens or lacinato kale, stems removed

1 tablespoon untoasted sesame oil or ghee

1 tablespoon black mustard seeds

Pinch of asafetida

Pinch of salt

Wash the greens and stack the leaves on top of each other. Cut the stems off. Roll tightly from one edge of the leaves to the other lengthwise, then hold one end and cut finely with a sharp knife to create long ribbons. Heat a large skillet on medium heat, add the oil and mustard seeds. Cook until they start to pop, less than a minute. Add the greens, cover with a lid, and steam for 1–2 minutes. Sprinkle with asafetida and salt to finish. Remove from heat and serve hot.

DOSHA NOTES

Ⓟ Use fennel seeds instead of mustard seeds.

Ⓚ Omit oil; steam the greens with a splash of water instead.

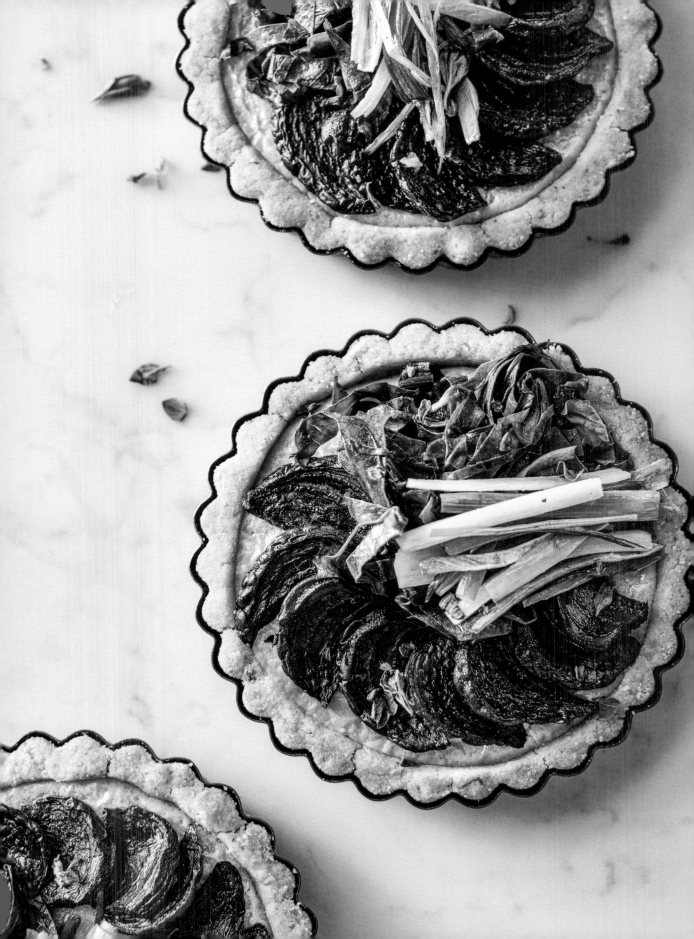

Savory Beet Tartlets

During the winter holidays, sometimes you want a dish that will wow friends and family. A switch-up from the regular dal-and-rice recipes, these beautiful beet tartlets are great for dinner parties or special events. Try golden beets or striped Chioggia beets for a more colorful presentation. If beets with tops aren't available, collards or kale make an easy swap for greens topping.

PREP: 45 minutes | COOK: 1 hour | YIELD: 6 servings

CRUST

3 cups brown rice flour

½ teaspoon salt

⅔ cup cold ghee or coconut oil

2 teaspoons fresh oregano, finely chopped

⅓ cup ice water

ROASTED BEETS

5 small beets with tops, trimmed, quartered, and cut into small ¼-inch slices

2 tablespoons olive oil

Pinch of salt

Fresh cracked black pepper, to taste

Place the brown rice flour and salt in a food processor and pulse to combine. Add the cold ghee or coconut oil and pulse until mixture resembles sand. Add the chopped oregano. With the food processor running, slowly drizzle in the ice water 1 tablespoon at a time, until the dough comes together to form a large ball (you may not need to use all the water). Remove the dough from the food processor and divide evenly between 6 small 4-inch tartlet pans greased with ghee or oil. Press evenly into the bottom and sides of each pan to make a thin ¼-inch crust. Use a fork to lightly prick holes into the bottom of each crust. Place in the fridge to set for 30 minutes. While the crusts set, prepare and roast the beets (recipe follows). Leave the oven on at 375°F when the beets are done, and then continue on to baking the crusts in the next step.

Remove the tartlet pans from the fridge and arrange on baking sheet. Bake for 15 minutes. Remove from oven and allow to cool before filling. Leave the oven on for the final step of cooking the filled tartlets (see page 282).

For the beets: Arrange the beet slices in a single layer on a baking sheet and drizzle with olive oil, salt, and pepper. Cover with parchment and bake for 20 minutes or until tender and a little crispy on the edges. Remove from the oven and set aside until ready to assemble.

continued

FILLING

2 cups macadamia nuts, soaked 1 hour

1½ cups water

4 tablespoons nutritional yeast

4 tablespoons lemon juice

2 tablespoons olive oil

1 teaspoon salt

1 tablespoon fresh thyme leaves

GREENS TOPPING

1 tablespoon olive oil

½ large leek, trimmed and sliced into 2-inch-long matchsticks (about 1 cup)

A couple pinches of salt, divided

2 cups finely cut beet greens

1 teaspoon lemon juice

For the filling: Drain and rinse the soaked nuts well. Combine all ingredients in a high-spend blender. Puree until creamy. Taste and adjust seasonings as needed. Set aside until ready to assemble.

For the topping: In a medium skillet, heat the oil and add the leek. Sauté on medium heat until tender. Sprinkle with a pinch of salt, reduce to low heat, and cook slowly for another 5 minutes, until lightly caramelized. Remove from the pan and set aside. In the hot pan, add the beet greens and stir until wilted, less than a minute. Sprinkle with another pinch of salt and lemon juice.

To assemble: Pour the filling into the baked tartlet crusts, each about ¾ of the way full. The filling will expand slightly once cooked, and you'll want to leave room to layer the beets and greens on top. Place the baking sheet of filled tartlet pans back in the oven and bake for 12–15 minutes. Remove from the oven and allow to cool for 10 minutes before carefully removing from the pans. Arrange the roasted beets, greens, and leeks on top of each tartlet. Serve warm.

DOSHA NOTES

(P) Use chard instead of beet greens.

(K) Use white beans instead of macadamia nuts.

Sesame Broccolini

For me, the best dishes are simple, easy ones you can quickly toss together that add tons of flavor and nutritional value to a meal, like this side of roasted sesame broccolini that can be added to any balanced bowl combination.

PREP: 5 minutes | COOK: 20 minutes | YIELD: 2 servings

1 bunch broccolini (about 8 florets)

2 tablespoons toasted sesame oil

1 teaspoon grated or minced fresh ginger

Pinch of salt

½ teaspoon sesame seeds

Preheat the oven to 400°F. Line a baking sheet with parchment paper. Trim the ends of the broccolini ¼ inch, keeping the stems long. In a mixing bowl, toss the broccolini with the sesame oil, ginger, and salt. Spread across baking sheet. Sprinkle the sesame seeds over the broccolini. Roast for 12–15 minutes, until tender and crispy.

DOSHA NOTES
Ⓟ Omit ginger.
Ⓚ Reduce oil.

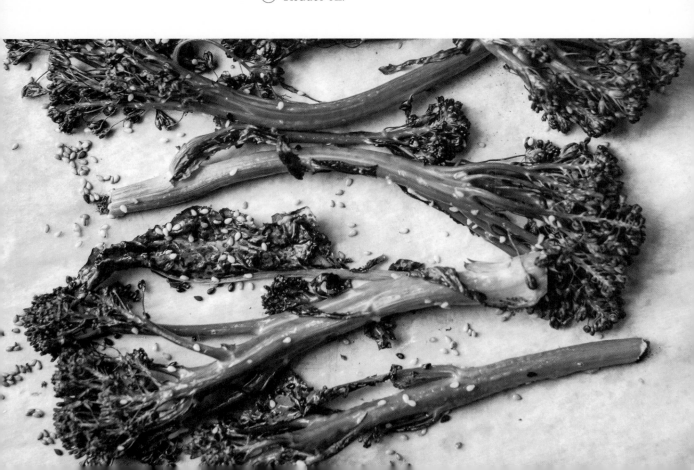

Chana Masala

This chickpea-based stew from North India is often quite spicy and served in a creamy tomato broth. This healthy alternative uses sweet potato and coconut milk to balance the pungent mix of spices. Dried mango powder, also known as amchoor powder, adds a unique tartness and little heat to the dish that balances both vata and kapha doshas.

PREP: 15 minutes | COOK: 90 minutes | YIELD: 4–6 servings

2 inches fresh ginger, minced

4 cloves garlic, minced

4 tablespoons ghee or untoasted sesame oil

1 tablespoon ground turmeric

1 tablespoon ground cumin

1 teaspoon ground coriander

½ teaspoon garam masala

½ teaspoon dried mango (amchoor) powder

⅛ teaspoon asafetida

2 cups sweet potato, cut into ½-inch cubes (about 1 large sweet potato)

5 cups soaked chickpeas (1½ cups dried chickpeas, soaked 8–12 hours)

2 teaspoons salt

1 tablespoon coconut sugar

Two 13.5-ounce cans of full-fat unsweetened coconut milk

4 cups water

5 kale leaves or collards, stems removed and roughly chopped

½ cup cilantro, stems removed and roughly chopped, plus 2 tablespoons for garnish

1–2 tablespoons lime juice

In a mortar and pestle, add the minced garlic and ginger. Grind until it becomes a thick paste. Set aside.

In a large pot, heat the ghee over medium heat, add the ginger-garlic paste. Cook for 1 minute until fragrant, stirring frequently to prevent burning. Add the remaining spices and cook for another minute. Add the sweet potato and chickpeas, stirring to coat in the spices. Cook for 5 minutes on low heat. Next, add the salt, coconut sugar, coconut milk, and water. Turn up the heat and bring to a boil. Cook for 20 minutes on high heat, then reduce to medium, cover with a lid, and simmer for 50 minutes, or until the chickpeas are tender. If using canned beans, note the cook time will decrease to about 30 minutes. In the last 5 minutes of cooking, stir in the greens and cilantro. Remove from heat and mix in the lime juice. Taste and adjust seasonings as desired. Garnish with cilantro to serve.

For a creamier variation, at the end of cooking, scoop 2 cups into a blender and puree until creamy. Transfer back to the pot and stir.

DOSHA NOTES

Ⓟ Use ¼ teaspoon asafetida in place of the ginger-garlic paste.

Ⓚ Reduce coconut milk and salt.

Winter Vegetable Biryani

Though you've likely found this dish in Indian cuisine, biryani actually comes from Persia and translates to "fried before cooking." While this healthier take on the classic recipe isn't fried, it does possess all the characteristics of a great biryani, with fluffy spice-scented rice laced with hearty vegetables, nuts, and herbs.

PREP: 10 minutes | COOK: 30 minutes | YIELD: 4 servings

WINTER VEGETABLES

½ head cauliflower, torn into small florets

2 cups cubed butternut squash or sweet potato

2 tablespoons olive oil

1 teaspoon garam masala

¼ teaspoon salt

Fresh cracked black pepper

BASMATI

2 cups dry white basmati rice, rinsed

3 cups water

¼ cup raisins

½ teaspoon ground turmeric

½ teaspoon ground coriander

4 cardamom pods

1 star anise pod

1 cinnamon stick

1 tablespoon rose water

½ teaspoon salt

1 teaspoon lime juice

GARNISH

Cashews or pistachios, pomegranate seeds, chopped cilantro, and yogurt

Preheat the oven to 400°F. Prep the vegetables and toss in olive oil, garam masala, salt, and black pepper. Spread the vegetables across a baking sheet. Roast for 30–35 minutes, until veggies are tender and crispy. Remove from oven and set aside.

For the basmati: In a medium pot, combine all ingredients, except the lime juice, and bring to a boil on high heat. Cover with a lid, reduce heat to medium-low, and simmer until the water is fully absorbed, about 15 minutes. Fluff with a fork and add the lime juice. Transfer to a serving bowl to combine with the roasted vegetables.

To assemble: Fold the roasted vegetables into the cooked rice. Sprinkle with cashews, pomegranate seeds, and cilantro. Serve hot. This also tastes great served with a dollop of fresh yogurt.

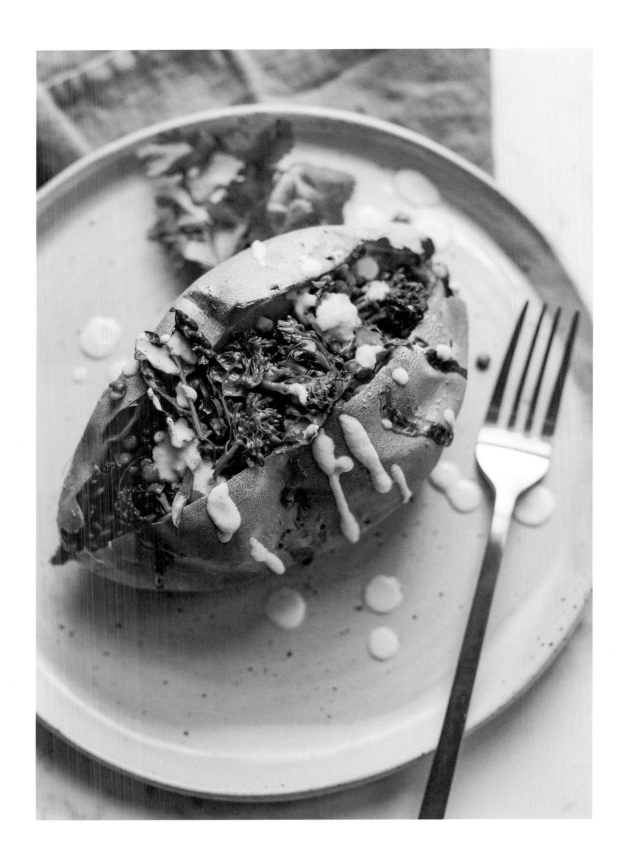

Mushroom & Lentil Stuffed Sweet Potatoes

How many ways can you use a lentil and keep it exciting? I've pondered this question while making this cookbook and looking at the many ways I use this versatile little legume. From soups and stews, to pancakes and salads—this savory lentil stuffing inside a slow-roasted sweet potato does not disappoint. With a little ginger, toasted sesame oil, and shiitakes, it departs from the Indian-influenced flavors of traditional Ayurvedic cooking while still nourishing and balancing the body in deep winter. A hot oven and long cook time are the secrets to really caramelized and delicious sweet potatoes.

PREP: 8–12 hours for soaking lentils | COOK: 75 minutes | YIELD: 4 servings

4 large sweet potatoes

1 cup French black lentils, soaked overnight

1 tablespoon minced fresh ginger

1 tablespoon minced garlic

2 green onions, minced

2–3 tablespoons toasted sesame oil

2 cups broccolini, cut into small florets

8–10 shiitake mushrooms, stems removed and chopped

4 lacinato kale leaves, stems removed, and cut into fine ribbons (chiffonade cut)

½ teaspoon salt

Fresh cracked black pepper

1 tablespoon lemon juice

Optional: cilantro, microgreens, for garnish

Optional: Sunseed Sauce (page 289) or dollop of yogurt, for garnish

Preheat the oven to 425°F. Scrub the sweet potatoes. With a fork, poke holes in each sweet potato. Wrap each potato individually in parchment paper and arrange on a baking sheet. Roast for 60–75 minutes, or until caramelized and tender.

Bring a small pot of water to a boil, add the lentils, and cook for 12–15 minutes or until al dente. If lentils are not soaked, the cook time will be longer. Avoid overcooking. Strain and set aside when done.

Mash the garlic, ginger, and green onion together in a mortar and pestle, or on your cutting board using a sharp knife. In a large skillet, heat the oil on medium heat, add broccolini, stir to coat, and cook for 2–3 minutes. Add the shiitakes, and cook for another 2 minutes. Add the garlic-ginger-green-onion mixture, and cook for 2 minutes. Cover with a lid to steam for another 2–3 minutes, until tender. Stir in the greens and cook until slightly wilted, less than a minute. Remove from heat, stir in the cooked lentils. Season with salt, pepper, and lemon juice. Set aside.

Remove the sweet potatoes from the oven. Slice each sweet potato lengthwise to create a slit down the center. Stuff with the mushroom-lentil mixture. Top with fresh cilantro or a handful of microgreens and a drizzle of sunseed sauce or a dollop of yogurt.

DOSHA NOTES

Ⓟ Omit garlic and green onions; substitute ⅛ teaspoon asafetida.

The Yogi Bowl

The Yogi Bowl follows the format of the balanced bowl (see page 158). It balances building and cleansing foods and incorporates the six tastes. Don't be daunted by the multiple steps in this recipe; with the right tools and prep, this bowl is easy to prepare and cuts down time on meal planning for a few meals. I make the grains in the rice cooker and use a pressure cooker to quickly prepare the beans. A quick steamed root vegetable, sautéed greens, a creamy dressing you can make for the week, and a spoonful of kraut completes this balanced macrobiotic-inspired tridoshic bowl.

PREP: 8–10 hours, for soaking beans and seeds | COOK: 1 hour | YIELD: 4 servings

ADZUKI BEANS

One 3-inch piece kombu

1 cup dried adzuki beans

2 tablespoons tamari

½ bunch cilantro, plus more for garnish

SIMPLE GRAIN

1 cup dried brown rice, millet, or quinoa

2½ cups water

Pinch of salt

KABOCHA SQUASH

1 small kabocha squash

For the beans: Combine the kombu and beans in a bowl and cover with 1 inch or so of water. Soak overnight. Drain the kombu and beans; discard the water. Slice the kombu into small strips.

Place the beans and kombu in heavy pot with lid—enameled cast-iron works best. Cover with water. Bring to a boil and cook uncovered for 10 minutes. Reduce heat to low, cover with a lid, and cook for 40 minutes, or until the beans are soft and tender. In the last 10 minutes, add the tamari and cilantro. The beans will become thick and stew-like. Remove from heat and serve hot.

Note: To reduce cooking time, use a pressure cooker to cook the beans and follow the pressure cooker instructions on cook time.

For the grain: Rinse well before cooking. In a small pot, combine the grain, water, and salt. Bring to a boil, cover with a lid, reduce heat to medium-low, and cook until water is fully absorbed and grains are tender. Serve hot.

For the squash: Cut the squash in half, scoop out the seeds, and remove the stem. Cut into 1½-inch-thick wedges. Arrange the wedges in a large skillet and cover with water. Bring to a simmer at medium heat and cook for 15 minutes, or until tender. Drain off the water and serve hot.

1 cup hulled sunflower seeds, soaked 1 hour

1 clove garlic

2 tablespoons ume plum vinegar

2 tablespoons lemon juice

1½ cup water

QUICK GREENS

1 teaspoon untoasted sesame oil or ghee

3 cups chopped kale, collards, chard, or spinach

Squeeze of lemon juice

TOPPINGS

Chopped cilantro

Kraut or kimchi

Sesame seeds

For the sauce: Drain and rinse the sunflower seeds. Combine all ingredients in a high-speed blender and blend until creamy. Store in a jar in the fridge for up to 3 days.

For the greens: In a skillet, heat the oil on medium heat and add the greens. Add a splash of water to steam. Stir a few times to coat in oil. Turn off the heat. Squeeze a bit of lemon juice over top and serve hot.

To assemble: Scoop a spoonful each of simple grain and adzuki beans into a bowl. Layer the greens and kabocha squash on top. Drizzle with sunseed sauce and, if using, finish with a garnish of fresh cilantro and sesame seeds. You can add any toppings you like; try adding a spoonful of kraut or kimchi to bring in the sour taste and spice up the dish. Serve hot.

Chocolate Date Scones with Maple Tahini Drizzle

Dessert for breakfast? These scones go either way. For a gluten-free variation, use the oat flour as the primary flour in the recipe and omit the spelt flour. The maple tahini drizzle also goes great on a bowl of breakfast porridge!

PREP: 10 minutes | COOK: 30 minutes | YIELD: 8 servings

SCONES

1¼ cups spelt flour

¾ cup oat flour

2 teaspoons baking powder

3 tablespoons cacao powder

½ teaspoon ground cinnamon

½ teaspoon salt

½ cup melted ghee or coconut oil

⅓ cup maple syrup

2 teaspoons vanilla extract

1 tablespoon orange zest

¼ cup cold water

6 Medjool dates, pitted and chopped

MAPLE TAHINI DRIZZLE

¼ cup tahini

¼ cup maple syrup

4 tablespoons water

Preheat the oven to 350°F. Line a baking sheet with parchment paper. In a bowl, combine the spelt flour, oat flour, baking powder, cacao powder, cinnamon, and salt. Fold in the melted ghee, maple syrup, vanilla, and orange zest. Pour the water into the batter and mix lightly, careful not to overmix, then gently fold in the chopped dates.

Using about ½ cup of batter per scone, space evenly across the baking sheet and use your hands to shape the batter into small triangles. You can also form the dough into a circle about 6 inches wide and 1 inch high, then use a knife to cut and divide into 8 triangles. Place in the oven and bake for 10 minutes. Rotate the baking sheet and place back in the oven for another 8 minutes. Remove from the oven and allow to cool for 10 minutes before serving. Drizzle the maple tahini sauce over top.

For the drizzle: Combine all the ingredients in a blender and puree until creamy. Store in an airtight jar in the fridge for up to 5 days.

DOSHA NOTES
(P) Swap carob powder for cacao powder.
(K) Skip the tahini drizzle.

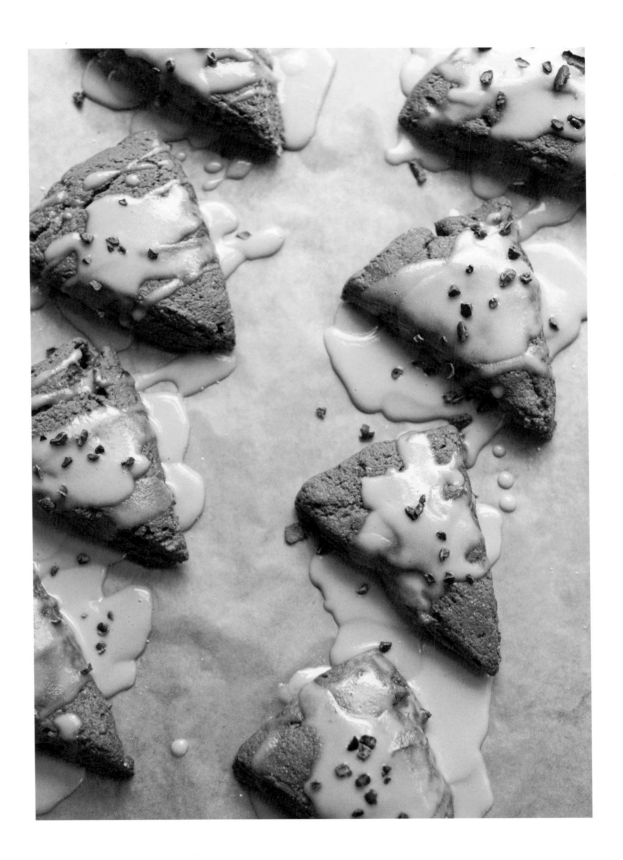

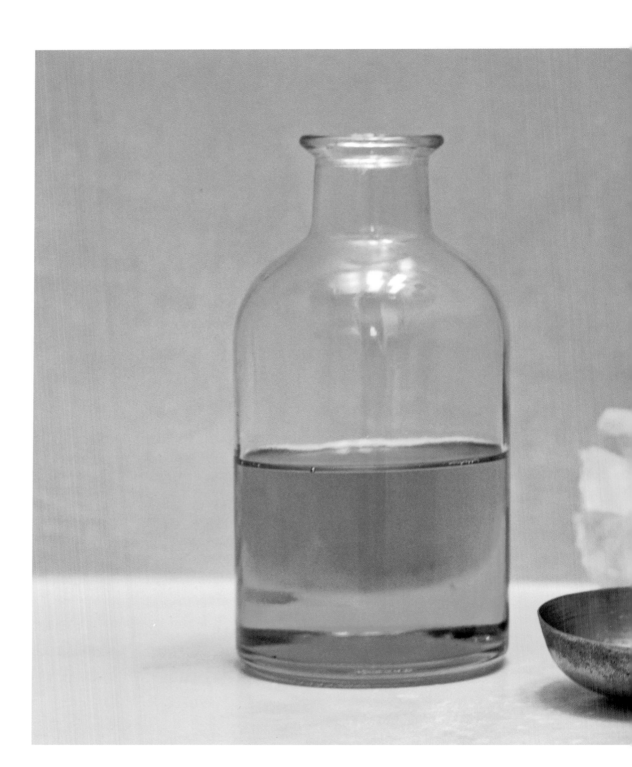

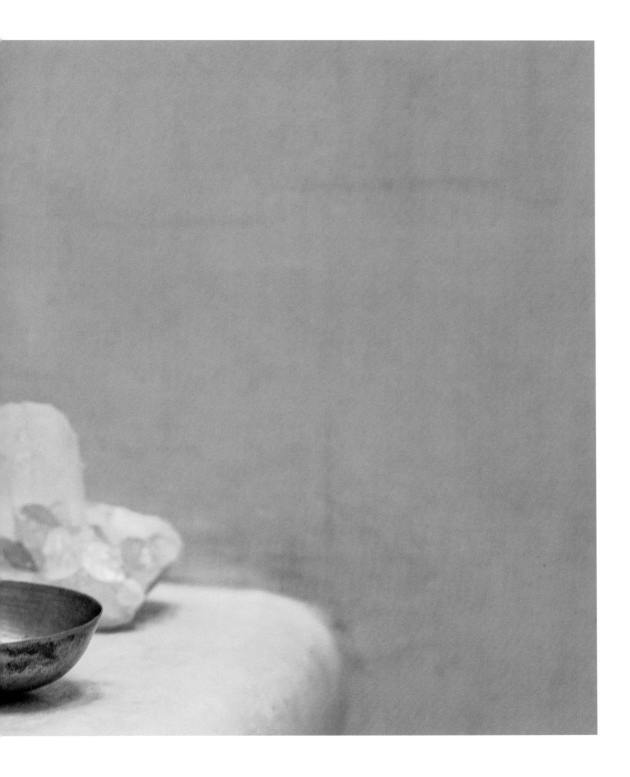

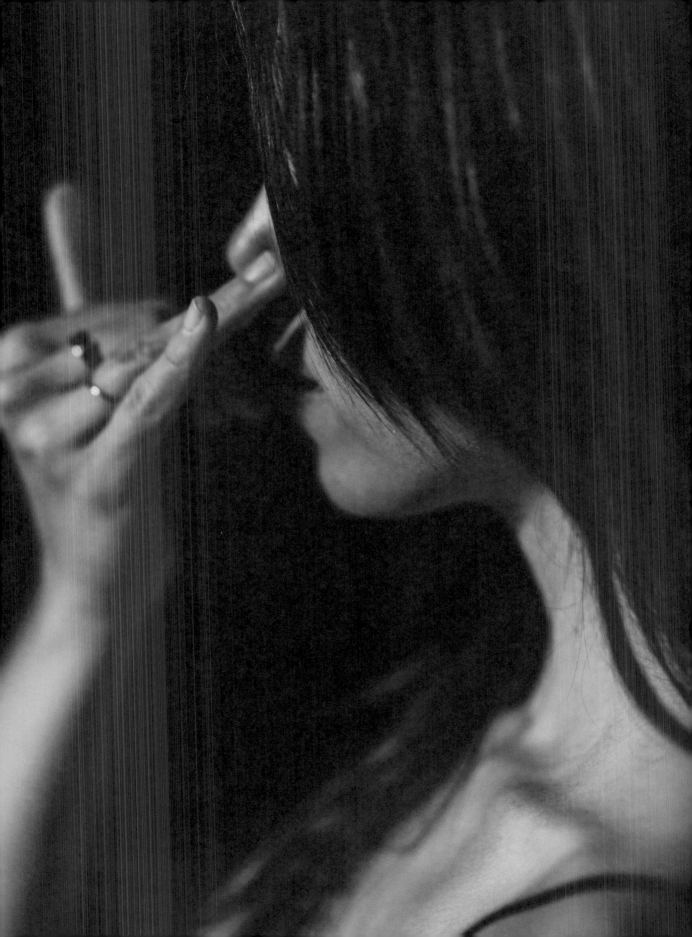

CONCLUSION

Inviting Grace into Your Year

My teacher once said that it's a good thing when you're being chiseled and polished by the challenges of life. Like a crystal with its many faces, when held to the light you can see the complexities that lie within, shaped by time and pressure. And when angled toward the sun, sometimes all those complex layers cast a brilliant rainbow, reflecting back the beauty in those challenges.

As I've reflected on how to end this book, one key word keeps coming to mind: *grace*. Grace is the special ingredient to navigating life with ease when difficulty arises. The greatest gift yoga and Ayurveda has given me is the ability to be malleable and remain stable in myself in challenging times. Stability is defined by how quickly we can rebound and return to neutral after being influenced by an external force or pressure. This is our real work, to have a fluid attitude and approach to nature's seasonal influences and life's curve balls while maintaining a daily practice that anchors us in clear seeing of reality.

Maybe your year didn't go as planned. Maybe you didn't cook as much as you wanted to or make it onto your mat at the same time every morning. *That's okay.* The beauty is that you have time. And the truth is, you are whole just as you are. Remember, this book is about embodying this wisdom on a very practical, very real, everyday level. Whether you follow the teachings to a T is not the point. Rather, it's about falling in love each day and making it your own living practice. Let this knowledge you've learned steep and mature through the seasons ahead. Return to it time and time again, with grace and a joyful heart.

ACKNOWLEDGMENTS

To Juree Sondker, Audra Figgins, Kara Plikaitis, and the whole Roost Books team for making this process not only possible but uplifting and fun each step of the way.

To Cassie Ballard, thank you for your tireless work as pitta project manager and creative partner on this book, for holding the vision and helping navigate us there. I couldn't have done this without you!

To my family—thank you, Dad, for always being in full support of my work. To my mom, thank you for introducing me to this path, for the giggles in the yoga studio as a kid, and the many meals, travels, and studies shared together that have shaped the contents of this book. And to my aunt, who gave me first kitchen job at age six and taught me passion for food and flavor.

To my incredible photography team—Ellie Baygulov, Cassie Ballard, Todd Scott Ballje, Lindsey Bolling, Joshua Diem, and Lora Villanueva of RNR Creative. Thank you for helping me bring the many visual aspects of this book to life.

To the sponsors and artisans who so generously donated their products, time, skill, and spaces for the book's production—Solare, Śūnyatā Sri Lanka, Salt & Water, Architectural Antiques, Makra Handmade Store, Magic Linen, Marissa Freeman Beauty, Chelsey Ann Artistry, Dillon and Kyle Tisdel, Chelsea and Matt Millunchick, Richard Spera and Casa Gallina, and to Karen and Majik for your brilliant natural plant-based dyeing and seamstress talents.

To my peer reviewers—Adena Harford Bright, Brianne Beauregard, Krissy Leonard, Emma Treharne, Christina Werthe, Erin Johnson—thank you for your invaluable knowledge and feedback that shaped this book.

To my friends and fellow authors who kept me sane along the way, shared their writing tips, and boosted me up with loving encouragement—thank you, Jessica Murnane, Heather Crosby, Laura Plumb, Laura Wright, and Almila Kakinc-Dodd.

To my recipe testers and kitchen team, it's your taste buds that made the recipes so special!

And to all my teachers and those who've walked this path before me, those who've devoted their lives in service to others and share the wisdom of the Vedas, I bow humbly to you with eternal gratitude.

REFERENCES

Frawley, David. *Yoga & Ayurveda: Self-Healing and Self-Realization*. Twin Lakes: Lotus Press, 1999.

Frawley, David. *Yoga for Your Type: An Ayurvedic Approach to Your Asana Practice*. Twin Lakes: Lotus Press, 2001.

Lad, Vasant. Textbook of Ayurveda. Vol. 1, *Fundamental Principles of Ayurveda*. Albuquerque, NM: Ayurvedic Press, 2002.

Meulenbeld, G. Jan. *A History of Indian Medical Literature*. Groningen Oriental Studies. Groningen, Neth.: Egbert Forsten, 1999.

Mohan, A. G., and Indra Mohan. *Yoga Therapy: A Guide to the Therapeutic Use of Yoga and Ayurveda for Health and Fitness*. Boston: Shambhala Publications, 2004.

Pisharodi, Sanjay. *Acharya Vagbhata's Astanga Hrdayam: The Essence of Ayurveda*. Vol 1. Self-published, 2016.

Sharma, Ram Karan and Vaidya Bhagavan Dash. *Caraka Samhita: Text with English Translation*. Vol. 1–7. Varanasi, Chowkambha Sanskrit Series, 2009.

Stiles, Mukunda. *Ayurvedic Yoga Therapy*. Twin Lakes: Lotus Press, 2007.

Svoboda, Robert. *Prakriti: Your Ayurvedic Constitution*. Twin Lakes: Lotus Press, 1998.

Tiwari, Maya. *Ayurveda: A Life of Balance*. New York: Healing Arts Press, 1994.

Tiwari, Maya. *The Path of Practice: A Woman's Book of Ayurvedic Healing*. Toronto: Wellspring/Ballantine, 2001.

Wujastyk, Dagmar, and Frederick M. Smith. *Modern and Global Ayurveda: Pluralisms and Paradigm*s. Albany: State University of New York Press, 2008.

RESOURCES

Kitchenware

www.ancientcookware.com // Traditional cookware

www.instantpot.com // Electric pressure cookers

www.bluebirdgrainfarms.com // Organic heirloom grains

www.korin.com // Japanese knives, suribachi, and steamers

www.makrashop.com // Artisanal clay cookware

www.nutrimill.com // Countertop grain mills

www.meliwraps.com // Reusable beeswax storage

www.vitaclaychef.com // Electric clay rice cookers

www.vitamix.com // High-speed blenders

Supplies

www.agnihotrasupplies.com // Agni Hotra ceremony kits

www.banyanbotanicals.com // Ayurvedic herbs, oils, cooking supplies, and online dosha quiz

www.biosonics.com // Tuning forks

www.livinglibations.com // Natural plant-based skincare

www.lotusbloomingherbs.com // Quality chyawanprash source

www.manduka.com // Quality eco-friendly yoga mats, props, and clothing

www.mountainroseherbs.com // Organic herb supplier

www.pureindianfoods.com // Ghee, spices, and cooking supplies

www.trihealthayurveda.com // Traditional Ayurvedic body oils and herbal jams

Programs & Schools

Ayurvedic Institute // www.ayurveda.com

Kripalu School of Ayurveda // www.kripalu.com

Mount Madonna Institute // www.mountmadonnainstitute.org

National Ayurvedic Medical Association // www.ayurvedanama.org

Wise Earth School of Ayurveda, Bri Maya Tiwari // www.wiseearth.com

Panchakarma Centers

The Arogya Center: Albuquerque, NM // www.thearogyacenter.com
The Ayurvedic Center of Vermont: Burlington, VT // www.ayurvedavermont.com
Purnam Center: Pomfret, CT // www.briannebeauregard.com
Dr. John Douillard: Boulder, CO // www.lifespa.com
Myrica Morningstar: Kauai, HI // www.ayurvedabliss.com
Vaidyagrama: Kerala, India // www.vaidyagrama.com

Further Reading

Acharya Vagbhata's Astanga Hrdayam: The Essence of Ayurveda, Volume 1 by Sanjay Pisharodi
Ayurveda: A Life of Balance by Maya Tiwari
Ayurveda Cooking for Beginners: An Ayurvedic Cookbook to Balance and Heal by Laura Plumb
Ayurveda: The Science of Self-Healing by Vasant Lad
Ayurvedic Yoga Therapy by Mukunda Stiles
Balance Your Hormones, Balance Your Life by Claudia Welch
Everyday Ayurveda Cooking for a Clear, Calm Mind: 100 Simple Sattvic Recipes by Kate O'Donnell
Practical Ayurveda: Secrets for Physical, Sexual and Spiritual Health by Atreya
Prakriti: Your Ayurvedic Constitution by Robert Svoboda
Yoga & Ayurveda: Self-Healing and Self-Realization by David Frawley
Yoni Shakti: A Woman's Guide to Power and Freedom through Yoga and Tantra by Dinsmore-Tuli

For more Ayurvedic living resources, visit www.vidyaliving.com/book to access
interactive cooking and yoga guides that bring your seasonal practices to life.

INDEX

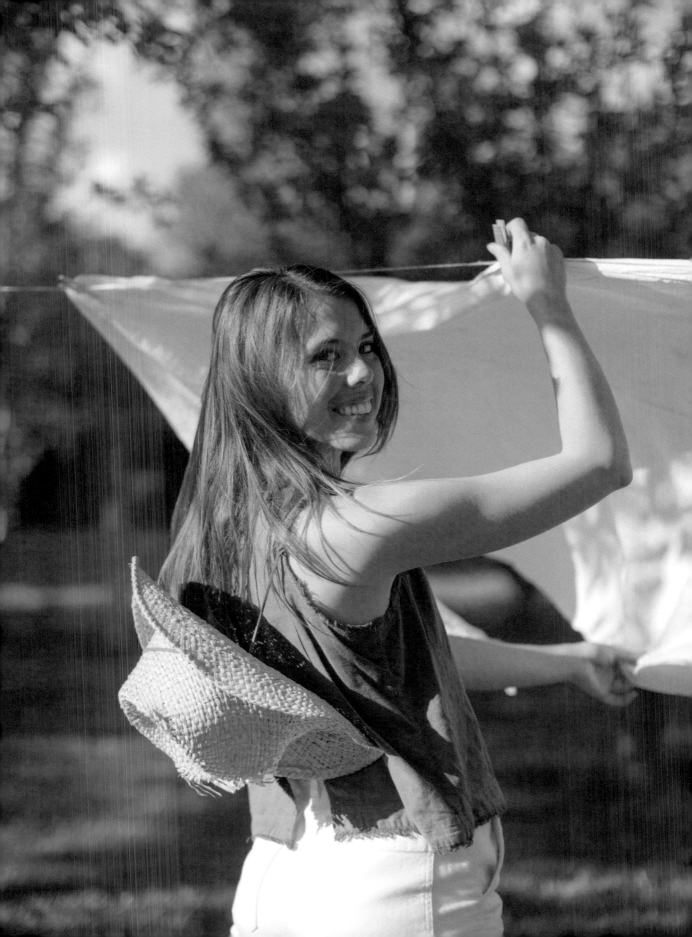

ABOUT THE AUTHOR

Claire Ragozzino is a certified yoga instructor and Ayurvedic counselor with a background in holistic nutrition and natural cooking. Her work is dedicated to bringing yoga, Ayurveda, and nutrition to a modern lifestyle. She is the author of the popular site, *Vidya Living*, and also writes and photographs for online and print publications surrounding topics of food, culture, and our relationship to nature. Claire works with clients around the globe and leads immersive workshops and retreats. Learn more about her work at www.vidyaliving.com.

Roost Books
An imprint of Shambhala Publications, Inc.
4720 Walnut Street
Boulder, Colorado 80301
roostbooks.com

Cover photo by Lora Villanueva
Design by Kara Plikaitis

9 8 7 6 5 4 3 2 1

First Edition
Printed in China

♾ This edition is printed on acid-free paper that meets the American National Standards Institute
Z39.48 Standard.
♻ Shambhala Publications makes every effort to print on postconsumer recycled paper. For more
information please visit www.shambhala.com.
Roost Books is distributed worldwide by Penguin Random House, Inc., and its subsidiaries.

Library of Congress Cataloging-in-Publication Data
Names: Ragozzino, Claire, author.
Title: Living ayurveda: nourishing body and mind through seasonal recipes, rituals,
and yoga / Claire Ragozzino.
Description: First edition. | Boulder, Colorado: Roost Books, an imprint of Shambhala Publications,
Inc., [2020] | Includes bibliographical references and index.
Identifiers: LCCN 2019048058 | ISBN 9781611807493 (trade paperback)
Subjects: LCSH: Medicine, Ayurvedic—Formulae, receipts, prescriptions. | Yoga. | Vegetarian cooking.
| Seasonal cooking. | LCGFT: Cookbooks.
Classification: LCC RM236 .R334 2020 | DDC 641.5/636—dc23
LC record available at https://lccn.loc.gov/2019048058